LOVE YOUR GUT

The Practical Guide to Sustainable Weight Loss from the Inside Out

SUE RITCHIE

TO THE READER

This publication contains the opinions and ideas of its author. It is intended to provide helpful and informative material on the subjects addressed in the publication. It is sold with the understanding that the author and publisher are not engaged in rendering medical health or any other kind of personal or professional services in the book. The reader should consult his or her medical or other competent professional before adopting any of the suggestions in this book or drawing inferences from it. The author and publisher specifically disclaim all responsibility for any liability, loss, or risk—personal or otherwise—that is incurred as a consequence— directly or indirectly—of the use of any applications of the contents in this book.

First edition published by Sue Ritchie

www.LoveYourGutBook.com

Copyright © 2015 Sue Ritchie

Sue Ritchie has asserted her right under the Copyright, Designs, and Patents Act, 1988, to be identified as the author of this work.

ISBN-13: 978-1517068677

Reviews of *Love Your Gut: The Practical Guide to Sustainable Weight Loss from the Inside Out*

'If you have been struggling with your weight for years and have wondered why you just haven't been able to be successful, well, this book explains why. Not only is the explanation simple and easy to understand, but Sue also shows you in a very practical, step-by-step way how you can address the root cause of your weight issue and transform your health from poor to amazing, ditching those extra pounds in a sustainable way.'

'So you can say goodbye to yo-yo dieting forever and hello to a vibrantly healthy and slimmer you!'

—Jennifer Gilchrist – Business and Personal Leadership Mentor

'Enlightening, thought provoking and engaging. Sue shows you a whole new way of looking at health, healthy eating, and shedding those extra pounds without starving or calorie counting. She presents a methodical and passionate, holistic approach to weight loss that works. It is compelling and easy to read'.

—Clive Wragg – Company Director

'Sue lays bare the mysteries of why gut health is such a big issue in today's world and how the way most people are currently eating is having a negative impact on their overall health and wellbeing. Packed with handy tips, practical advice, and an innovative approach to weight loss, her Your Ecstatic Health Eating Plan blows away the myth that healthy eating has to be bland and boring'.

—Mary Jane Boholst – Successful Networking Mentor

Table of Contents

About The Author

'The doctor of the future will no longer treat the human frame with drugs but rather will cure and prevent disease with nutrition.'

—*Thomas Edison*

S UE RITCHIE WROTE THIS BOOK so that you to could take your health to a whole new level of vibrancy. She totally believes in a holistic approach to health, taking into account mind, body, and spirit. Sue also believes that the key to good health lies in prevention through loving and taking care of your body with good nutrition.

Four years ago, Sue found herself in what she calls a 'black hole', where she was unfulfilled, unhealthy, overweight, and putting up with Hashimoto's disease, which is an auto-immune disorder. Her journey to great health was kick-started by making two big decisions that pushed her out of her comfort zone. The key factor for Sue was making those decisions by listening to her heart and honouring her value. Therefore, Sue invested in the personal development help that she needed to start her journey out of that black hole. She also had to get off of the treadmill and give herself quiet time.

Had Sue Ritchie not taken those actions, she would not be in the place she is now, doing what she says is the best job in the world: helping *others* to get great health too.

Foreword

DEAR HEALTH- AND WEIGHT-CONSCIOUS PERSON,

If you've been feeling 'out of sorts', tired, listless and more, but can't put a finger on why, you know you have an auto-immune disorder. If your weight refuses to shift despite trying all kind of 'diets', then you're about to discover an astonishing explanation that will completely and utterly change your life in a way that you cannot imagine.

LOVE YOUR GUT - The Practical Guide to Sustainable Weight Loss from the Inside Out is the answer you've been looking for to deliver an exciting and new vibrancy to your life and living through improved health and weight loss. This book is NOT another diet book. Sue Ritchie will hold your hand through a process that will revolutionise the way you eat; this not only improves gut health, but it also induces weight loss without conscious 'dieting' because YOUR body will no longer crave foods laden with sugar, carbohydrates, and gluten.

Is it impossible to believe a life without cakes, biscuits, pasta, and chocolate? Take a look at the testimonials, and notice that every one of Sue's clients has said exactly the same thing . . . It is true; the most ardent cake queen is now body clean, no longer even wanting the sugar- and gluten-laden foods.

Let Sue guide you to *LOVE YOUR GUT*, shift some pounds, and live your life with greater energy, vitality, vibrancy, and purpose.

Your healthy future depends on it!

—Raymond Aaron
New York Times Best-Selling Author
www.2dayTycoon.com

(Raymond is the author of Branding Small Business for Dummies and Double Your Income Doing What You Love, besides many other bestselling books. He is known as the #1 success and investment coach, teaching people just like you how to use his goal-setting strategies to change your life.)

Dedication

THIS BOOK IS WRITTEN FOR all of my readers who find yourselves in that place of being stuck in your life and feeling helpless about your health and wellbeing. You are feeling as if nothing can help you achieve the changes you want regarding your health and weight issues.

A few years ago, I was in that exact same place, so I know how you are feeling. I want you to know that there is an answer that will help you to take your health and wellbeing from poor to amazing. That is the reason I have written this book, so you too can transform your health.

Love to you all,
Sue Ritchie

Acknowledgements

MY THANKS GO TO THE Universe for the gift of Hashimoto's auto-immune disease. This occurrence led me on a path of research and self-discovery that ultimately resulted in my receiving a 'Cosmic Fax' that gave me the answers to my health and weight issues. I was then able to heal myself and transform my health from poor to amazing. My life is now truly blessed, and I have the best job in the world in helping other people, who are struggling as I was, to transform their health and their lives from a place of being stuck to being amazing.

I want to give a huge thank you to Linda Curtis, my special friend, for your constant and invaluable support, encouragement, and help along the way. Thanks also to my wonderful husband for putting up with my being closeted away writing and my not being as present in your life as you might have wanted over the last 3 months.

Thank you also to Vishal Morjaria, my book architect, for your guidance and advice along the way and also for ensuring that my book made it to the printers and publication on time.

My book also wouldn't have been the same without the hard work of James Zarrello, who had the task of taking my book and whipping it into shape by eliminating any errors.

—Sue Ritchie

CHAPTER 1

How You Can Take Your Health From Mess To Success

'Most people have no idea how good their body is designed to feel'.

—*Kevin Trudeau*

I WOULD LIKE TO START BY congratulating you for taking your first step on this journey of taking control of your health by buying this book. I know that is a HUGE step to take. So I would really like you to truly appreciate how amazing you are in making this decision.

You see, I know from my own experience that you taking this initial step is going to open up so many other doors and opportunities in your life. By getting your health into a great

1

place, you are going to start to feel amazing, and your energy levels are going to grow. I know that when you feel great, things will start to change for the better in your life, your relationships, and your work. This is because you have started to value yourself in a way that you haven't before.

So are you feeling really frustrated with the situation you are in? I know I was. I'm betting that you have probably tried all sorts of things to shift those extra pounds. Did you find that they either didn't work or, if they did, you only lost a few pounds initially? Then, you found that when you stopped and went back to eating the way you did in the past, those pounds just piled on again.

I know how that feels because two and a half years ago, I was two and a half stone (35 lbs) heavier than I am today. I had been like that for too many years to remember. The incredible thing was that I always ate healthfully by government nutritionists' standards all my life. So, on that basis, I was following a good diet, and I was exercising regularly. But no matter what I did, I just couldn't lose that weight. I had really gotten to the stage where I thought, What the hell, I'm going to have to stay this way for the rest of my life! I had come to the point of pretty much accepting that.

One of the reasons I wrote this book is because I know that it doesn't have to be that way. And I want to show you how you can lose those excess pounds, without starving and calorie counting, and keep those pounds off for the long term.

Another reason I wrote this is because it really upsets me when I hear so many women saying that they have low energy, health, and weight issues. Then, when they go to visit the doctor, they often hear things like 'What do you expect? It's just your age'. Many doctors just don't seem to have any answers or strategies to offer. Or if they do, it will probably involve prescribing some form of drug. In reality, in most cases it's something we just don't need. It's as if we have to put up with feeling like rubbish for the next thirty or forty years, and we can't expect to live our lives to the fullest from now on. How crazy is that?

You see, I know it doesn't have to be that way, and we do have a right to feel full of energy and be vibrantly healthy well into our seventies and eighties. It also upsets me to see so many people nowadays just accepting the idea that low energy and poor health is just something they have to put up with and get on with. That to me is terribly sad. And I know that it doesn't have to be that way.

There is an answer to changing this situation, so I am making this my big mission to get out there into the world and share what I have learnt from my own personal experience with as many people as I can. There is a root cause to this situation. And if you are really willing to do what it takes to address it, then I can promise you that you too can achieve sustainable, ecstatic health and transform your life. How great would that be? Is this something that you would want?

To me, great health is a totally holistic thing. As human beings, we are made of a total system that includes our bodies, our minds, and our emotions or spirit. So if all of these elements are not in a good place, then we cannot achieve great health because they all affect each other. The food we eat affects how we feel emotionally. If we are not getting the right nutrition, vitamins, minerals, and fluids into our bodies, this will have an effect on the way our brains work and also how we feel emotionally. And if we don't feel good mentally, it affects how we go about our day and how we interact with other people. It also affects our productivity. In fact, it affects every aspect of our lives.

So if you are thinking, Well, that's all very well for you, but it can't be possible for me, please trust me that it is all possible for you. I want to share briefly with you my story because I feel it will be useful for you to know that I was in a place two-and-a-half years ago, where perhaps you are now. Today, however, I have kept off the 2.5 stone/35lbs that I lost two-and-a-half years ago, and there has been no yo-yoing of my weight. My energy levels are great, I feel healthy every day. I have had no colds, flu, coughs, or any viruses since I addressed the root cause of my weight and health issues. I enjoy life and live it to the fullest.

So first let me take you back to 5th July 2009. If you were with me on that day, you would have seen me sitting in my doctor's surgery waiting for the results of a blood test. You would have heard the doctor say 'As I had suspected, the blood test is showing that you have Hashimoto's disease'. 'Okay' I said, 'What does that mean?'

The doctor explained that it was an autoimmune disorder where the body attacks the thyroid gland, making it underactive. Now I have always had an interest in alternative health and nutrition, so I knew something about autoimmune disorders. So I asked the question, 'If it's an autoimmune disorder problem, there's got to be a way that I can correct it and get myself back to normal, right?' The response from the doctor was 'Oh no, that isn't possible. You are going to be on medication now for the rest of your life'. However, I wasn't ready to accept that. So over the next few years, I spent a lot of time—hours and hours—doing research, reading books, and reading articles online to really learn more about autoimmune disorders, and particularly the one I had, Hashimoto's disease.

There is, however, another part of my story, which really plays an important part in this whole situation of getting my health into a really good place. You see, I was brought up to believe that you had to work really hard to be successful. So for most of my corporate career, I worked long hours, and I juggled looking after my partner, the home, and then having children. I had senior corporate marketing roles that involved my working long hours, and I also travelled abroad too. Then, I started my own direct marketing business 15 years ago. The idea of doing that was to work less and be able to spend more time with my children. That worked for a couple of years, but soon the business started to grow. I then began to employ people. And guess what? The long hours started to creep back in a big way.

Four-and-a-half years ago, I found myself in a very dark place. I was working hard but not seeing the financial reward for my time. I was unfulfilled, and you could even say that I was just existing rather than living. And I had a number of other health issues along with Hashimoto's disease. I was overweight, and I suppose I was at that point where I was coming to accept that I would never be able to lose those extra pounds. There wasn't a lot of fun in my life. There never seemed to be any time for that. All the things I had loved doing I let go in my life because I was so focussed on having to be working in my business. In fact, you could say I lived to work rather than working to live.

I had gotten to the point where I knew that something in my life was going to have to change, but I really just wasn't sure how that could happen. I felt totally helpless at the time. I always had this negative voice in my head that told me that I wasn't good enough. I also had a voice that told me I wasn't very good at communicating with people. But then someone introduced me to a programme that really enabled me to start turning my life around. Interestingly enough, and to my great surprise, I learnt that everybody has a negative voice in their head. And this negative voice likes to keep us safe and secure. But the problem is that it stops us from putting ourselves out there and achieving all that we want to achieve in our lives.

I also learnt that as a woman, I had always lived my life more in the masculine. It was always about being busy and taking action all the time, and I realised that this lifestyle hadn't really served me that well at all. You see, as I stepped more into the feminine and also allowed myself to have time to do the things that I enjoyed, my life really started to improve. I started on that journey to make my way out of what felt like a dark cave and really started to allow the real me to emerge slowly more and more.

One of the key things for me during my change was taking time out to meditate every day. I took time for walks in nature. I started to spend time focussing on myself and healing myself. Then what happened next was—and I know this might seem quite incredible—but I received what I can only call a 'Cosmic Fax'. Now you might be wondering what that is. Well, the only way I can explain it is to say that some words just popped into my head. It wasn't a thought. Instead, the words just appeared. This gave me the answer as to why I couldn't lose weight and why I had health issues. The message told me that the root cause of my health and weight issues lay in my gut health.

The key factor in my gut health was a problem with Candida. Now I am sure that when you hear this word, you probably immediately think of thrush, particularly if you are a woman. Or, perhaps—as a couple of people have said to me when hearing the word—that artificial sweetener stuff! You may now be thinking, Well I haven't got a problem with thrush, so this is not going to be relevant for me. The thing is, Candida is not only about having bouts of thrush. It goes much deeper than that as you will find out later on in the book.

On receiving that information from the 'Cosmic Fax', I started to research all about Candida and found the process for eliminating it. Part of that process was to adopt a whole new eating plan. The result was that the pounds fell off me, my energy levels soared, and the health conditions that I had disappeared over time. Now you can imagine that being able to achieve this had an amazing impact on my life and my relationship with my husband. Everything also changed with all of my family and friends. This new eating plan basically allowed me to start enjoying my life to the fullest.

There were some really important things I learnt from my four-year journey out of the black hole I was in. I would like to share those with you because I know that if you can take these on board, they will help you greatly on your transformation journey to a new, healthier you.

The first really important thing to remember is that you must truly value yourself. You deserve to invest time and money and address your health since you are truly worth it. In addition, if you look after your own health, then you will be able to look after your family better. You deserve to take time out for yourself to do the things you love. You will feel so much better for it, and you will be more productive as a result. You will also be building the foundation for a healthier life during your old age too by taking control of your health situation now. This is better than just crossing your fingers and hoping that you will be healthy in the future.

Why is that we tend to look after our cars better than our own bodies? We make sure to put the right fuel in our cars, we check the water, we have them serviced regularly, and we check the tyres and oil. Why do we do this? We do it because we know that if we don't, we could be on a journey and the car might break down. Now that would be a real nuisance, wouldn't it? What a hassle that would be to have to call roadside assistance and try to get home or get to our destinations without the car if it couldn't be fixed there and then.

When it comes to our bodies, though, so many of us are okay with putting the wrong fuel in, not topping up the water, not having a regular MOT (annual road safety check), and over-revving the engine continuously. Then we just cross our fingers and hope that somehow we will keep going. Is this correct?

Staying healthy is fundamental to being able to really enjoy life to the fullest. Indeed, we should really all be able to enjoy our lives to the full. Life shouldn't be a constant struggle of hard work. It is about keeping a balance between work and fun but also doing what we love.

The second key thing I learnt was that taking time to slow down has some amazing benefits. Get out and have walks in nature, spend quiet time doing nothing. Start meditating every day. It will help you feel calmer to deal with the stresses and strains of everyday life, and you will become more creative and more productive. I know it may seem counterproductive, but believe me, it really works!

The next thing to do is really something that I had a serious problem with: asking for help. Don't be afraid to ask for help. Asking for help doesn't mean you are a failure but is actually a sign of great courage. After all, we can't do everything on our own; we do need support and help from other people. This is something I have had to really take onboard and practice. You see, I always felt that if I asked somebody for help, I was admitting that I had failed in some way. But isn't true at all.

That negative voice may be popping up now and saying to you that this is going to be too difficult for you. It's saying that you're never going to be able to lose weight because you've tried before and you've never succeeded. So what makes you think this is going to work for you now? Please stop listening to this negative voice. It's there to keep you 'safe and secure', but it really stops you from taking your life to a whole new level. Tell it that you don't need its advice. Tell it you are going to be okay and you can do it.

You might feel that you are unhappy or you are stuck in your life, and I know how that feels. It doesn't feel great, and you might feel totally helpless. You may be thinking that it really isn't possible to make the changes you want to make. However, I want you to know that it is possible. If I was able to do it, and my clients are able to do it, then you can too. I am going to give you practical guidance and tools through this book that will mean it can all happen for you if that is what you truly want.

What I also need to emphasise is that this is a journey. It isn't a quick fix even if you think that is what you want. You will know deep down that quick fixes haven't worked before. I know, because like me, you probably have tried some quick-fix diet plans. You may have found that they worked only for a short period of time.

However, to keep your weight down in a sustainable way and keep your health in a great place, these other plans haven't delivered. Central to what I will share with you in this book is how to lose that weight sustainably without starving, struggling, calorie counting, or just eating a lettuce leaf! This can be achieved because we will get to the root cause and address this issue that is preventing you from losing weight.

My clients are getting exceptional results when they follow the process I have devised. On average, people are losing at least one and a half stone (21lbs) to two stone (28lbs) in a 90-day period. They see their energy levels and health and wellbeing soaring as well. My clients are also reaping additional benefits as the program has had a positive transformational effect on their entire lives. This step by step process will unfold for you over the following chapters.

Before we move on to the next chapter, I would like you to do an exercise. I know it is tempting to just keep on reading and get to the end of the book, but I would really encourage you to stop and do the exercise since it will be beneficial to you.

9

Exercise: To get started, find yourself a quiet place where you won't get disturbed. Then get a piece of paper and a pen or pencil. Ideally, you want to spend about half an hour thinking about this.

This exercise will also will provide a great opportunity for you to start practising setting aside quiet time just for you.

I'd like you to sit and start thinking about what you want from your life in the future.

Really think very deeply about this and dream big about it. Don't put any blocks or limitations on what you want.

Now paint a detailed picture of how you would like to look physically.

What clothes would you like to be wearing?

How would you like to feel every day?

What would you like to be doing?

What and who would you like to have in your life?

Where would you like to live?

What sort of lifestyle would you like to be living?

What do you want from a health point of view?

Think about the near future, but also think about how you would like your health to be later in life.

You can write this all down, but I would encourage you to truly go into the detail of what your life would be like and how you want to feel. Start imagining what it would feel like to have that life and be actually living it.

You could also create a pictorial collage using images and words that fit with how you want your life to be so that you have a visual image of your desire. So get the scissors, magazines, and glue out, and have fun doing it too!

Then keep that reminder in a place where you can see it every day.

You can access free bonuses at
www.loveyourgutbook.com

CHAPTER 2

Is The Devil In Your Diet?

'You are what you eat—so don't be fast, cheap, easy, or fake'.

—*unknown*

Is the Devil in your diet? Well, that is an interesting question, isn't it? I wonder what you are thinking having read that question? In fact, it would be good for you to ponder the question for a few minutes because you may find the answer all on your own.

There is one thing, however, that is of real concern to me. Most of us just never stop to listen to our bodies, for if we did, we would probably stop eating certain foods. We would do this because we would have realised by the way our bodies feel that a particular food or foods are not doing us much good.

- Do you find that your stomach feels bloated after eating bread, for instance?

- Do certain foods give you indigestion?

- Do some foods tend to have an impact on your bowels?

- Are there foods that leave you feeling hungry and craving for more?

The problem we are seeing is that most people's diets have changed significantly over the last 20 to 30 years. It used to be meat and two vegetables back in the day when food was lovingly cooked from scratch. Now, however, as lives have become increasingly busy, many people just grab for something that can be prepared and eaten as quickly as possible. They buy ready meals that can be hurriedly placed in a microwave or an oven to save time, or they buy frozen-food items that can quickly and easily be cooked. This sort of speedy meal is also being fed increasingly to children since we have to rush them off to school and then after-school activities. The problem I see is that we are doing this without thinking about the potential long-term impact on our children's' health.

If we don't take care of what our children are eating today, this is going to have an impact on their health as they get older. So eating well when you are young is an investment for future health.

The problem with processed and ready-prepared meals is that they have already been cooked once, and then you heat them up again in an oven or microwave. After all of that processing and cooking, I wonder how much nutrition is left to be absorbed by your body. You then must recognize that for the food to be kept 'fresh', most brands have chemical ingredients added as well as sugar, salt, and even yeast to improve the flavour. Most of these ingredients make for just dead calories, but more importantly, they can have negative effects on our health.

Then there is the increased incidence of people either eating out or grabbing takeaway meals for quickness. In this scenario, many people's diets are increasingly based on eating only protein and carbs. Somewhere in the mix, vegetables seem to have disappeared even though they compose a critical part of our diets by providing valuable vitamins and minerals. Along these lines, it really annoys me that when you are eating out in many restaurants, the price displayed is for a dish that consists of meat or fish with chips or potatoes of some kind or rice. But then you have to pay an additional price if you want to have vegetables with your meal. It really should be the other way around. The price should be for the meat and vegetables, and then if you want the carbohydrates, you pay extra for those!

It is very difficult today to find a snack meal for lunch that isn't wheat based. But with my clients, I am seeing their health improve dramatically by removing gluten from their eating habits. This is because many do not tolerate gluten very well as part of their diet.

In the Western world, we seem to be falling out of love with the whole concept of eating and enjoying the process of preparing food and eating it. We seem to be increasingly losing sight of what eating food is all about. Why is that?

To me, the real reason for this is that we are have become so caught up in the daily 'time' trap of never having enough hours to do all the things that we need to get done. As a result, eating now is a low priority activity in our lives. For many people, it becomes a case of merely grabbing the nearest thing and getting it into our stomachs quickly to satisfy our hunger pangs. We are not thinking about the impact of the food choices we make. We don't realize that these choices could be seriously impacting our health and potentially shortening our lives. More importantly, our food choices are having a major impact on the quality of our lives.

You see, the saying, 'You are what you eat' is really true. The food you eat will impact not only your body but also how you feel emotionally and mentally. In fact, what you eat can make you feel depressed, irritable, and grumpy. It can also make you prone to anxiety and more susceptible to feeling stressed. On the other hand, eating certain foods can make you feel happy and calm. Either way, your diet will have a major impact on the health of your gut. So why is that important?

The change in our diets in the Western world, where we predominantly tend to eat protein and carbohydrates and also foods with high sugar levels, means that our bodies are becoming increasingly acidic.

Foods such as protein, carbohydrates, and sugar are acid-forming substances in the body. This can also include many fruits too. Strangely enough, though, lemons—which you might think are acid forming—actually form alkaline in the body. Vegetables are also alkaline forming in the body.

Meanwhile, foods such as meat, cheese, milk, fish, eggs (especially the yolks), grains, and carbohydrates increase acid levels in the body.

In addition, medications, soda pop, processed meat and foods, artificial colours and flavours, and preservatives and sugar make us more acidic.

At this point, I expect you to be asking, 'So why does this modern-day change in our eating habits matter?'

Well, it matters because our bodies function best at a neutral Ph value of about 7 to 7.4. So if we have too acidic a body, health problems start to arise.

When our bodies are too acidic, it has an impact on our bones, teeth, muscles, joints, connective tissues, various organs, and other bodily systems. It causes extra stress to be placed on the body, which then can have a further negative effect on many health issues.

When the body has to work especially hard to reduce and buffer extra acidity, it can have the following effects on our health:

- Obesity, slow metabolism, and inability to lose weight

- Yeast/fungal overgrowth

- Weight gain, obesity, and diabetes

- Slow digestion and slow elimination

- Reduced ability to absorb minerals and other nutrients

- Bladder and kidney conditions, including kidney stones

- A weakened immune system

- Reduced ability of cells to repair themselves

- Osteoporosis, weak or brittle bones

- Joint pain and aching muscles

- Chronic fatigue and generally low energy

- Mood swings

- Premature aging

To maintain optimal health, our diet should consist of 60% alkaline-forming foods and 40% acid forming.

Alkaline-forming foods are generally green vegetables, some

fruits, peas, beans, lentils, spices, herbs, seeds and nuts. Conversely, acid-forming foods are generally meat, fish, poultry, eggs, grains and legumes.

So to start changing the alkalinity of your body, you should eat a higher proportion of vegetables every day, focus on eating alkaline-forming foods, and reduce the number of acid-forming foods in your diet.

You can access a bonus chart of alkaline- and acid-forming foods at www.loveyourgutbook.com

Another factor that is impacting the acidity of our bodies is that most people are just not drinking enough water every day.

Research has shown that around 80% of the population is walking around each day dehydrated. But in reality, we need to be drinking around 2 litres of filtered or mineral water a day plus other fluids. One of the problems with dehydration is that it produces the same feeling as being hungry, so all too often we think we are hungry and grab a packet of crisps, a chocolate bar, or some other snack instead of drinking a glass of water.

Another problem is that when we are feeling thirsty, our bodies are already dehydrated. If we are not drinking enough water every day, we cannot dilute the acidity of our bodies, which then compounds the problem. So a very simple way to start making an impact on the acidity of your body is to start drinking lots more water on a regular basis throughout the day.

Handy Health Tip

When you feel hungry, instead of grabbing something to eat, go and get yourself a glass of mineral or filtered water and drink that first, and then see how you feel afterwards.

There is another factor that is having a major impact on our health, and is contributing to poor gut health. This is the entire issue around stress. So many people are living their lives in a constant state of stress. I certainly suffered with stress very much in my life until I learnt to take my foot off the pedal and allow myself more quiet time.

When our bodies are stressed, it causes cortisol to be released into the bloodstream, yet cortisol is a form of sugar. So this chemical change adds to the acidity imbalance in our bodies. Stress is supposed to occur during a flight-or-fight situation that is over in a fairly short space of time. But what is happening to many people today is that the stress button is continually 'on' over a long period of time. That means that the body doesn't have time to recover, and this puts pressure on your adrenal system, which in itself can cause health issues.

Apart from making healthful eating choices, you can also help to manage your stress levels by meditating every day. In today's society we are driven to be connected 24 hours a day. As a result, we are always checking social media, e-mails, and texts or are on the phone constantly throughout the day and late into the evening. This happens so much that it is very difficult for us to 'switch off'.

This over-connectedness then has a knock-on effect because if we don't switch off for a period of time—particularly before going to bed—it becomes very difficult to sleep well. Lack of sleep then has a knock-on effect on our health and wellbeing, so we get caught in a vicious circle.

It is important for your wellbeing and also your creativity to take quiet time out in your life. That means being just at one with yourself and your own company. A great way of getting that quiet time is to make meditation a part of your normal daily routine. I'll be talking more about the benefits of quiet time later on in this book.

If you have never tried meditation before, I highly recommend that you get started with this bonus. If you do currently meditate, or you have in the past, then this meditation exercise will also help you start the journey to a healthier, slimmer you.

You can access a free bonus: a guided meditation and a chart showing you which foods are acidic or alkaline forming in your body at www.loveyourgutbook.com

CHAPTER 3

The Surprising Connection Between Gut Health And Weight Loss

'Take Care of your body. It's the only place you have to live'.

—Jim Rohn

S O HOW COULD THE STATE of your gut health make you overweight?

Being overweight is about eating too much, not exercising enough, and eating the wrong foods, isn't it?

Well, yes, they do all have a part to play. However, there is one element that is missing, and that is the importance of gut health to our overall health. I struggled for years being overweight and even when I was eating 'healthfully' according to good nutrition guidelines.

I was doing regular exercises, and I wasn't eating huge amounts of food. But nothing I did made a difference until I found about the importance of gut health in this equation.

Did you know that approximately 70 to 80 percent of your immune tissue is located within your digestive system? That means your gut essentially is your immune system. That is the reason why gut health is so important.

The gut is often the first entry point for exposure to pathogens (bad bacteria and viruses that can cause disease). Therefore, your gut immune system needs to be thriving and healthy in order for your body to avoid illness.

As I mentioned in Chapter 1, it wasn't until I received that 'Cosmic Fax' that told me the answer lay in my gut health and I found out that the real problem was Candida overgrowth in my body that anything changed for me.

So what it is Candida? I expect that most of you know because of the condition known as thrush that it causes. Candida, though, is a bigger issue than just having a bout of thrush. Yet many people have not heard of the other health issues that it can cause.

Candida albicans (although there are other forms, this is the main one) is a type of yeast. As such, it is a normal part of the microbes that live in your gastrointestinal tract—your gut.

Small amounts of the yeast also live in various warm, moist areas throughout the body, including the mouth, rectum, vagina, and parts of your skin. Its numbers are naturally kept in check by the good bacteria and other microorganisms that make up your microbiome, which is the community of microorganisms that inhabit your body. Problems, however, arise when that natural balance of good bacteria and microorganisms gets disrupted.

Candida has a job to do in aiding digestion and nutrient

absorption in our bodies, but it becomes a problem for us when it gets out of hand.

So how does this disruption in the natural balance of the flora and fauna in your gut happen?

Well, it is partly due to the high sugar, high carb eating we seem to have adopted in recent years in the Western world. This trend is significant because our bodies are increasingly acidic based on the way we are eating.

But there are also some other factors that have resulted in gut health being a problem for many people today.

One of those additional factors is the prescription of antibiotics.

How many times have you been prescribed antibiotics in your life? It has probably been many, many times. Have you found yourself suffering from a bout of thrush after taking antibiotics?

The frequent use of antibiotics has an impact on our gut health because they kill all the good bacteria in our gut as well as the bad. This outcome then disrupts the natural balance of good bacteria in our gut needed to sustain good health. The body consequently undergoes an imbalance in gut flora and fauna, and then poor health issues start to appear. For this reason, it is always a good idea to take a course of good probiotics immediately after you have completed a course of antibiotics. Even better would be to avoid antibiotics altogether unless taking them is absolutely necessary.

If you are a woman, the use of contraceptive pills also has an impact on your gut environment, making you more susceptible to Candida overgrowth in your body.

When the good bacteria have been destroyed, this enables the growth of Candida to get out of hand as there is nothing there to hold it in check anymore. In addition, the fact that Candida thrives from sugar and refined carbohydrates intensifies the problem. In fact, sugar and carbs are Candida's favourite foods. To make matters worse, if we are stressed all the time, we are releasing lots of cortisol into our bodies, and that is another form of sugar. So the cortisol boost is just providing more food for Candida to keep growing strongly. Happy days!

Once Candida gets into overgrowth status, it starts to move out of the gut and into other parts of the body. Have you ever had athlete's foot? This is—as you probably know—a fungal infection, and it is caused by Candida.

When Candida moves into other parts of the body, a myriad of other health problems start to emerge. Many of the symptoms may seem like very minor things, and most people don't tend to worry too much about them. They tend to creep up on us over time, so we have a tendency to regard them as sort of 'normal' and just accept them.

A key factor of Candida overgrowth and how it impacts the inability to lose weight is that it starts to break through the gut wall. This then causes 'leaky gut syndrome'. When this happens, food particles escape from the gut and get into the bloodstream. Of course, food particles shouldn't be in the blood, so this problem causes an immune response and inflammation. Such bodily malfunction is a root cause for the growing number of people who have food intolerances. The key ones tend to be gluten and dairy.

Once you have a leaky gut, you are then not able to absorb all the vitamins and minerals that your body needs to keep it healthy. Your body always wants to be operating at its most efficient level so that it can keep the bodily control centre—your brain—working effectively. This problem then has the effect of making you want to eat more so that your body can extract the same amount of nutrition that it needs. So the leaky gut issue explains why you want to eat bigger portions of food.

But that is not the only factor. When you are eating many processed foods—which have sugar, salt, and yeast typically added, as well as other chemicals—these also have the effect of making you want to eat more food as well.

So how do you know if you have a problem with Candida overgrowth in your body?

Here is a list of the key symptoms of gut-health problems:

- Problems focusing and concentrating, brain fog, memory problems

- Digestive problems/bloating/wind

- Athlete's foot/fungal nail infections

- Cravings for sugar and carbohydrates

- Irritability, mood swings, anxiety, or depression

- Feeling tired all the time/suffering from chronic fatigue, fibromyalgia (chronic, widespread pain)

- Autoimmune diseases such as Hashimoto's, rheumatoid arthritis, MS, ME, vitiligo (loss of skin pigment) , Crohn's (bowel disease)

- Skin problems such as eczema, hives, rashes, itching

- Vaginal infections, thrush, recurrent cystitis (bladder infection), rectal or vaginal itching

- Seasonal allergies, such as hay fever or itchy ears

- Food sensitivity or intolerance

- Pain and/or swelling in joints (stiffness in the mornings)

- Abdominal pain

In my case, I had trouble with thrush in my early twenties and then would invariably have a problem after taking a course of antibiotics. From time to time, I suffered with athlete's foot and also digestive problems with wind on a regular basis.

Then, in more recent years, I struggled with not being able to focus or concentrate, and this was impacting the way I worked in my business. I was even having memory issues. This is especially telling because I've always had an excellent memory. I used to be able to remember hundreds of books by their ISBNs— the unique numbers on the back of each book that identifies them—when I worked in publishing in my early career. This is sad, isn't it? It got so bad that I was having situations where I 'knew' I had recently held a particular document. I thought I knew where I filed it, but when I looked it up, it wasn't there.

There were times when I felt that I must have been going mad. It was scary and frustrating. Is this something that happens to you?

I also had a handful of very frightening moments when I was driving, where I just seemed to lose all awareness of where I was and where I needed to turn. It was as if my mind got scrambled. Luckily, these situations didn't turn into any accidents, and these were odd moments. Thank goodness my driving has been totally accident free. Have you had any moments like that? Do you find that you are having regular 'minor accidents' in your car?

I also kept having recurring issues with breathlessness and feeling I couldn't get enough air into my lungs. I'd get sent off to the hospital, but the doctors couldn't find any reason for it. In case you are thinking I am a hypochondriac and have a tendency to bring these illnesses on, I can tell you that I just hate being ill because it stops me from being active and doing all the things I need and want to do. And anyway, my 'hard work script' will have me dragging myself to work even though I am really not well enough!

I also suffered with digestive problems, had cravings for sugar and carbs, had itchy ears, and had food intolerances to dairy and gluten.

I also know from my own family situation that if you suffer from Candida there is a likelihood that other members of your family may suffer from it as well. I believe that some people are more genetically predisposed to having a problem with Candida overgrowth than others.

Unfortunately, both my mother and father had passed away before I found that root cause for myself. But I do believe that had I known this when they were still alive, they could certainly still be with me today. My son had similar difficulties, so we addressed his problem at the same time I addressed mine.

Exercise

I would encourage you to read the above list of symptoms and then think about your body. Some of the symptoms you may think of as being 'normal' to you, particularly if you have had them for a very long time in your life. We tend to accept these things as just being 'the way it is'.

- Write down the ones you think you have.

- How long have you had some of these symptoms?

- Depending on your age, it would be a good idea to think back to when you were younger, too.

- Have you had some of these symptoms in the past?

- Are you struggling with staying focused? Do you feel that your brain is somehow foggy?

- Have you had problems with thrush a number of times in your life?

- What about athlete's foot?

As well as taking note of the symptoms and being aware of the types of foods you are eating, you can also do a simple test to see if you have a problem with a Candida overgrowth in your body. This is called 'the spit test'. It isn't foolproof, but does give you an indication.

All you need to do is take one-half of a glass of clear water up to bed with you at night, and then before you do anything in the morning, take a mouthful of water. Hold the water in your mouth, swish it around, and then spit it back out into the glass.

The saliva will float. Then leave it for 15 minutes, and look for the 'tails' hanging down from the top as shown in the diagram below. If within 15 minutes you see thin, tail-like pieces or strings extending downward into the water, this is a positive sign for Candida.

Other positive indications might be very "cloudy" saliva that sinks to the bottom of the glass within a few minutes or particles that slowly sink or suspend below the saliva glob. You are seeing colonies of yeast, which band together to form the strings.

If you do observe this, then Candida overgrowth is present in your body. But don't worry because something can be done about it. I will be addressing that process in future chapters.

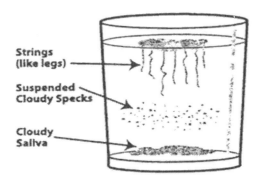

If you are not sure about your results, send me your photo of the glass side on when you have completed the test. tlc@yourecstatichealth.com

You can access free bonuses at www.loveyourgutbook.com—Check them out.

CHAPTER 4

Why Sugar And Carb Cravings Are Not Your Fault

'If you think everything is someone else's fault, you'd be wrong. If you think everything is your fault, you're also wrong. Assigning blame can keep you stuck in the problem. Move on to solutions'.

—*Sue Fitzmaurice*

S ONE OF THE THINGS that has held you back from really taking control of your health and weight issues been this dread of not being able to eat those sweet things that you seem to love? Do you just love those desserts, cakes, biscuits, chocolates, sweets, and ice creams? Does it feel like an addiction?

You know that those things need to go if you want to truly address your weight issues, but it feels like you would rather chop your arm off than stop eating those things. Can I see you nodding 'Yes'? You see, I know that many people feel like this is such a big issue for them that they just don't bother to tackle their weight problem. It just seems to be too big an issue to overcome.

Do you feel as if it would be just total deprivation for you if you couldn't have those things?

Given the choice of savoury foods, what would your choice be? What would you choose off the menu at a restaurant?

Would it be a pizza, a nice pie, sandwiches, a pasta dish—like lasagne or spaghetti Bolognese—or chips? Is there a desperate need for you to consume a lot of carbohydrates? Moreover, is toast your food of choice for breakfast? And do you tend to choose things made with refined white flour?

Well, if your answer is 'Yes', I totally understand how you feel.

What if I told you that those cravings are not your fault? How would that make you feel? Would it make you feel a little better about yourself? Would it allow you to let go of some of the pressure you are putting on yourself when making your eating choices? The fact that you are pressurising yourself will not help you to release the weight you are carrying either.

I expect that you are now saying that this can't be true and are thinking, I crave these foods because I am weak willed, and I am addicted to them. I would encourage you to let go of that thinking, because it is being driven by things that are going on inside your gut.

In reality, when your gut is not healthy, and you have a problem with Candida overgrowth, this condition can drive the cravings that you are feeling for sugary foods and also refined carbohydrates. The reason for this is that Candida thrives on the sugar and the refined carbohydrates that you are consuming, so it becomes a vicious circle. The more sugar and refined carbohydrates you eat, the more you feed the Candida, and the more it then impacts your gut health and your overall health. And then you crave more sugar and more refined carbohydrates.

Also, when our gut health is not in a good place, we are not able to absorb all the vitamins and minerals that our bodies need for good health.

If you already have a Candida overgrowth problem in your body, and you eat or drink foods such as bread, beer, distilled spirits, and many processed foods that are made with yeast, you are just adding to the problem. Your body will be very sensitive to foods containing yeast, and this will exacerbate your health problems. The next time you are out shopping, check the ingredients on processed foods. What is listed on their package labelling?

One thing that I know is once you go through the process of eliminating the Candida overgrowth problem, and you heal your gut, you will find that you no longer crave or even want sugary foods.

At this stage, I know you will be thinking that this is really unbelievable. I understand that you think this way now. The same was true for most of my clients who went through my 90-day programme. Almost everyone thinks this way at the time they start on the journey. But they now know that they will no longer have those cravings since they healed their gut and changed the way they ate. So I encourage you to hold this space for yourself.

When they start my programme, and we talk about the sugar and carb craving situation, they ask me 'When I have finished the programme, will I be able to go back and eat the way I do now?'. My answer is always, 'You won't want to go back and eat the way you do now, because you will feel so great, both physically and mentally. Your body will simply no longer want those foods that you crave now'.

All of them come back to me at the end of the programme and say 'Sue, you know when I asked about going back to eating the way I used to when I started your programme, and you said that I wouldn't want to? Well, you were absolutely right because I really don't want to eat the way I used to anymore. I have no desire to do so at all because I feel so great'.

Are you really ready to do whatever it takes to get your health into a great place? Or are there some fears that are coming up for you? When we start to move towards the need to make changes in our lives, there are often fears that come up for us. This is perfectly normal and okay.

Whenever we start to move out of our comfort zones, we begin to feel uncomfortable and triggered. The problem is if we don't move out of our comfort zones, nothing in our lives is going to change. I am nonetheless pretty sure that what you do want is for changes to occur in your life so that you can live better and healthier.

Whether or not you have tried to lose weight in the past, or if you are looking to do this for the first time, there will fears that will come up for you right now. The following fears might be ones that you are feeling right now:

1. I am not going to be able to do this. I failed before, and I will fail again. I don't want to be a failure.

2. If I make this change for myself, it will affect the other relationships in my life, and I can't control that, so that makes me fearful of the unknown.

3. If I lose the weight, and my body shape changes, some of my friends might be jealous and not like me anymore.

4. My husband/partner fell in love with me when my body shape was as it is now. If I lose the weight, he might not fancy or love me anymore.

5. If I lose weight, I am going to become visible, and that makes me feel scared.

There may be other fears that come up for you, but I want you to know that whatever they are, they aren't real. Fears are only in our minds, and they just stop us from achieving the things that we really want to achieve in our lives. They can be overcome. Just make the reason why you want to do this big enough.

I'd like you to think of a time in your life when you had fears about something, but you decided to just go ahead and do it anyway. How did you feel about it afterwards? I am pretty certain that you'll say, 'It wasn't nearly as bad as I thought it was going to be'. The fear was actually worse than actually doing the thing you were afraid of.

I remember when I was 12, and I was doing my Personal Survival Swimming Silver Award. One of the requirements to gaining the Silver Award was to jump off the top board in the swimming pool. I have always been afraid of heights, and to some extent, I still am today. However, I really wanted to get that award. So there I was, standing on the top board. I stood there for what seemed like ages, having that 'discussion' in my head. One part of me was saying, Go on, you can do it. Just close your eyes and jump. But the other side was saying, Oh no, I'm scared! I really don't want to do this. Back and forth the argument went, over and over again. You know how that process goes!

Then finally, I just said, "One, two, three!" And I jumped and went for it. It seemed like forever before I hit the water. But once I had done it, I was saying to myself, That wasn't that bad at all. Why was I so scared? There was not a lot that could happen to me except land in the water and swim, so what was I scared of?

This is why I say that fears are not real. They are just in our minds. They purport to keep us safe and secure, but they just stop us from growing and experiencing new—and more often than not—better things in our lives. Fears hold us back from achieving success and making the changes we want and need in order to put our lives in a better place than we are today.

One thing I know for sure is that when we know we want something different for our lives, we just need to take that one small step in the right direction to start. Then we will see other things start to shift and change in our lives for the better. All too often, we allow those irrational fears that feel so real to us to stop us from taking the initial small step. Yet it is that first small step that will get us really moving into a truly better place for ourselves. We have to let go and trust because if we do, everything will work out fine. If you feel in your heart that this is what you want to do, then everything will be fine. There is nothing to fear. You will look back in a few weeks' time and wonder why you were so scared to make that initial step towards your better future.

So don't let your feeling that there is no way you can stop having sweet foods prevent you from making a start and getting your health to a better place. Your future self will thank you for feeling the fear yet being brave and doing it anyway. Then you will feel full of energy, and your health will be in a far better place. The added bonus is that you can look forward to having an active life full of fun and enjoyment as you get older.

So let's jump off the high diving board together and look to get your health in a great place. I will be metaphorically holding your hand, so you are not alone.

If you feel that you would like support on this journey, then you can find out more about some opportunities to get this at www.loveyourgutbook.com

CHAPTER 5

The Route To Taking
Your Health To Wealth

'Believe you can, and you're halfway there'.
—*Theodore Roosevelt*

I N THIS CHAPTER, I AM going to show you in a practical, straightforward way the things that you need to do to start eliminating the Candida overgrowth from your body and healing your gut. You need to follow this process for 90 days, but I can assure you will not want to go back to eating the way you do currently after you have gone through this process.

If you are taking any medications, or have health conditions, you should consult with your doctor before starting this programme. You must not rely on any information in this book as an alternative to medical advice from your doctor or other healthcare provider. If you have any specific medical questions about a medical matter, you should consult your doctor or other professional healthcare provider.

This is a totally natural approach, so there are no drugs involved in this process. You will, however, need to be taking some vitamins and natural supplements as part of the procedure.

I want to make the start of this journey to health as easy as possible. That is why we are not going to jump straight into eating differently. That would be stressful for you. Instead, we are going to take the slow wind-down approach into the process proper to get you slowly adjusted to the new way you are going to be eating.

You may be starting to hear that negative voice speaking to you and telling you that it is not going to be possible for you to follow this and be successful. If this is the case, I would encourage you to tell that negative voice that you really don't need its advice. You know exactly what you are doing, and you are going to be absolutely fine. You should say, 'I am going to succeed because I really want to. I am going to succeed because I totally deserve to because I am worth it'.

The principles of my approach are listed below.

You are going to be totally removing the following foods from your diet after the first 2 weeks:

1. Gluten

2. Sugar in all its forms as well as artificial sweeteners

3. All processed foods

4. Yeast

5. Dairy products (products made from goat's or ewe's milk can be consumed)

I bet you are thinking, So what am I going to be eating, then?

Please don't worry. It isn't as bad as you at first think it will be. You will be eating plenty of healthful, natural, quick-to-prepare, and tasty foods. You aren't going to be hungry or starving at all. I can assure you of that. What is more, they are all foods that the whole family can enjoy. I would encourage you to cook the same foods for the whole family. They will then be enjoying huge health benefits as well.

We have become conditioned into thinking that the way we are currently eating is the only way and that any other way must mean we will be consuming boring, uninteresting, and bland foods. This, on the contrary, is not the case. I would therefore encourage you to keep an open mind about this matter.

I know that it might seem as if taking sugar in all its forms out of your diet is a really big thing. I understand how you feel about that. You are not alone on this one. Most of my clients are concerned about how they will manage at the beginning when they work with me on my 90 -day programme: 'Bust through your weight barrier, boost your confidence, and supercharge your success'.

However, are you a person who used to take sugar in your tea or coffee? If your answer is 'Yes', then I ask you to think back to how you felt about not having the sugar in your tea or coffee the first time. You would have thought, I don't know if I am able to drink this. But when you stick to it, it will actually be alright as you get used to it. Then, after a few weeks, you are at a friend's house, and he/she offers you a cup of tea. Not knowing that you don't use sugar, they put some in. You then take a sip and then go, 'Ugh!' Is that right? This is because having tea with sugar now doesn't taste very nice anymore. Well, the same thing will happen when you remove sweet foods from your diet. In the end, you will not want to go back to eating them.

I know you don't believe me right now. That's okay. But hold your mind open, and trust me, because in a few weeks' time you won't want to go back to the way you are currently eating again.

There are very good reasons why these foods need to be removed from your normal diet. The key reason is that in order to kill off the Candida overgrowth, we need to remove the foods that feed it. The greater benefit that you are going to see is that your energy levels are going to increase and you are going to start to feel genuinely healthy in both body and mind. And you will be surprised at just how much the feel-good factor will start to impact other areas of your life and bring in some amazing opportunities.

You see, the food we eat has an impact on our brains, and therefore, on how we feel emotionally. It affects the way we react to situations. When we have a lot of sugar in our bodies, it can make us more prone to anxiety and also make us grumpy and short tempered. So if something goes wrong, we are likely to react badly to that situation instead of just taking a calm approach.

Wouldn't you like to be able to deal calmly with things that don't go your way rather than getting all anxious and upset?

Another reason for removing certain foods from your eating plan is that you may have intolerances that you are not even aware of. These issues could be having a negative effect on your overall health.

Admittedly, you will need to adjust your mindset a bit and keep in focus the end result that you so desperately want. So bring back the vision of what you want for yourself, and keep firmly in mind what you created when you read the first chapter of this book.

Whenever you feel that you might not stick your new diet plan, remind yourself of that vision of the healthy, slim, energised you. Just think about all the things you will be bringing back into your life and how good that is going to feel. Think about the lovely clothes you will be able to wear and how great you will feel, knowing that you look great.

The first thing you need to do is start getting prepared for this amazing journey to great health that you are about to embark on.

Clearing Your Food Cupboard and Fridge

To make this process as simple as possible for you, I have listed all the things that you need to be ready. Put a tick against each item as you complete it.

1. Prepare your food-storage cupboard by getting rid of the following things:

   All of your wheat-based breads, biscuits, cakes, snacks, sweets and chocolates. It might seem harsh, but take heart—over the next few weeks, your need for sugar, cakes, and biscuits will disappear even though you might find that hard to believe at this moment in time. You will also need to get rid of any ready meals and other processed foods.

   You can give these away or throw them away or maybe donate them to a food bank. That way, you are not wasting the food.

2. Review your refrigerator and ensure that you remove any food that is mouldy or is going mouldy. Then give it a really good, thorough cleaning.

3. Throw out any out-of-date spices, seeds, and nuts.

4. Discard old oils and all margarines/spreads. Substitute margarines/spreads with goat's butter. You will be doing your whole family a favour. You can use up what you have in stock over the first 2 weeks.

5. As for food storage, make sure that you have good, clean airtight rubber-sealed or preserving/storage jars available for storing nuts and seeds and other loose products that you are going to be eating. These items are good for storing your seeds and nuts in as well as loose foods such brown rice flakes, etc. The reason why they need to be airtight is that we need to prevent moulds from growing on the products. This can happen if foods are not stored in an airtight environment. Undoubtedly, food that has mould growing on it will just add to the problem of gut health.

   The small airtight preserving jars are ideal for storing your Crunchy Munchy Seeds, when you have made them. They can then be kept on your desk or taken with you if you go out. That way, you have a nutritious snack on hand whenever you need one. You can find the recipe for these in Chapter 6.

   Also, make sure you have glass containers for storing cooked food in the fridge. Plastic ones are okay, but glass ones are healthier because the plasticisers in the plastic can leach into foods. If you store leftover food in plastic containers, do make sure it is cold before you put it into the container.

6. You will need to buy the products that are itemised under the heading 'Shopping List' that you will find in Chapter 6 if you don't already have all of these. Furthermore, if you do have some of them and you have had them in your store cupboard for several

months and haven't used them, I would recommend that you throw them out and buy fresh.

7. I would recommend that you buy organic vegetables. These can be bought at most big supermarkets these days and some health food shops or organic farms, or you can arrange box deliveries on a weekly basis. These are great options as the produce will be nice and fresh.

   If you have an allotment, and you grow your own vegetables and don't use pesticides, then these are great to continue eating. It is not essential to buy organic vegetables, but I would recommend them. Non-organic foods are grown with the use of pesticides, and residues of the pesticides can remain in and on the food. So do make sure, if you are not using organic produce, that you wash your vegetables well first.

8. Where possible, it would also be best to buy organic meat. You could research on the Internet for a local organic farm, or there are those that deliver via mail order. Again, this is not essential. I know that budgets may not stretch to the additional cost. You will find, however, that once you get into the new way of eating and have all the new staples in your store cupboard, your normal weekly shopping spending will go down. So later on, you may feel that you can afford to start buying organic produce.

There will be a number of foods that you will be avoiding as part of the Your Ecstatic Health Eating Plan™, and I have listed these out below in as much detail as possible for you. It is essential that you do not consume any of these whilst going through this 90 day process.

Foods to Avoid

Sugars

Sugar in all its forms and foods that contain sugars should be eliminated from your eating plan.

These include the following:

- Honey

- Molasses

- Maple syrup

- Sugar substitutes/sweeteners – saccharin, aspartame, any branded artificial sweeteners, etc.

- Lactose from milk products

- Alcoholic and soft drinks even if they say they are sugar free

- Fruit sugar—This means no fruit either fresh or tinned

- Chocolate and sweets, even ones that say they are sugar free; these will have artificial sweeteners.

- Agave nectar/stevia

- Rice syrup

- Coconut sugar

- Palm sugar

- Fructose and glucose

Yeast

Yeast is found in a wide range of foods, particularly processed foods, along with sugar.

These include the following:

- Breads

- Cakes and Biscuits

- Marmite and other yeast spreads

- Pastries

- Stuffing mixes

- Products coated in breadcrumbs; for example, Scotch eggs, fish fingers, breaded chicken, chicken nuggets, breaded fish, etc.

- Mushrooms

- Soya sauce and tamari sauce

- All cheeses, particularly hard cheeses (soft goat cheeses that do not have a rind are okay)

- All types of dried fruits—raisins, sultanas, currants, dates, apricots, bananas, pears, figs, etc.

- All fermented drinks—beer, spirits, wine, and cider; no alcoholic beverages

- All malted products; you need to avoid any product that contains malt.

- All vinegars—except for apple cider vinegar

- Miso, tempeh, and tofu

- All smoked meats and fish, processed meats—ham and salami, etc.; they all contain yeast and sugar.

- Foods need to be fresh, so you do need to be careful about storage time in the fridge.

- Nutritional supplements that are not labelled as being yeast and lactose-free

Nicotine and Stimulants

- Coffee, black tea and green tea; this also includes decaffeinated coffee or tea.

- Cigarettes and cigars, nicotine supplements, and e-cigarettes

Refined Carbohydrates

All refined carbohydrates should be avoided. This includes all white flour, white rice, pasta and the things that they are used to be made into—bread, cakes, biscuits, scones, pancakes, etc. You should only eat the carbohydrates that are in the shopping list provided.

Gluten

Gluten is found in wheat and other grains such as rye, barley—and to some extent—oats. Many people are gluten intolerant without realising it. Gluten-free oats are okay to eat.

Margarines and Spreads

Hydrogenation is a process used to solidify vegetable oil in the manufacture of margarine. This technique damages fatty acids and undermines our health, so margarines are to be avoided. If you prefer to have margarine instead of butter, then Vitaquell, which is available in health stores, is fine to eat as it is doesn't use the hydrogenation method.

Goat's butter is a great alternative and can be bought in most large supermarkets. It is also a natural product.

Dairy

Replace cow's milk, (that even includes 'lactose-free' cow's milk) with either goat's or sheep's milk or almond milk. Almond milk is a great alternative to cow's milk as it has all the nutrition of cow's milk plus more. In fact, it has more calcium than cow's milk. Cow's milk yoghurts can be replaced with goat's yoghurt or coconut yoghurts.

You need to follow the instructions below for the first 2 weeks:

Week 1.

1. Start the morning before you have anything else with a cup of hot water and a slice of lemon. Cut a slice of unwaxed/ organic lemon, and place into a mug. Add some cool, filtered water so that it just covers the lemon, and then pour over hot boiled water. Give the lemon some prods with a spoon or knife so that you release some of its juice.

2. Before showering, dry brush your skin. This is a great process to help your body to detox. You can access a detailed description of how to do this on www.LoveyourGutbook.com. You should start to make this part of your daily showering routine.

3. Start to reduce the amount of sugar that you are consuming each day, but do this in a gradual process

over the next 2 weeks. Eat fewer cakes and biscuits and sweet things than you normally do. If you take sugar in your tea and coffee, then reduce the amount of sugar that you use. For example, if you usually have two teaspoons of sugar, then cut that by half, etc.

4. If you need to snack during the day, then replace sweet snacks with some nuts.

5. Reduce the amount of bread that you eat. If you normally have a sandwich for lunch, then try having a salad a couple of days a week in the first week. Then in the second week, make it 4 days. This should be vegetables rather than a pasta salad.

6. Start to reduce the number of processed foods that you are consuming. Cut down on ready meals, pizzas, etc., as much as you can.

7. If you normally drink a lot of tea and coffee that has caffeine, then start replacing some of these cups with herbal tea or a glass of filtered/mineral water instead.

8. If you typically drink a lot of fizzy drinks such as Coca-Cola, lemonade, other fizzy drinks, squash, etc., then start to reduce that as well and replace them with filtered or mineral water or herbal tea. You can put a slice of unwaxed lemon or lime into the water to add flavour, if you prefer.

9. Start to increase the amount of water that you drink each day. You should try to ensure that you are drinking at least 4 pints a day by the end of the second week. A great tip is to put a big jug of filtered/mineral water on your desk when you start work in the morning. Fill up a big glass, and drink that through the morning.

10. Increase the amount of vegetables that you have with your meals.

11. Each evening, before you go to bed, start writing in your notebook 5 things that you are grateful for during your day. This can be quite difficult at first, but don't worry if you can only manage 2 or 3 to start with. You will get better with practice. Try to focus on the small things that have happened in the day, and look for the positives in them. Also, if there are negative things have happened, try and see if you can find a positive in it anyway. For example, what could you learn from the experience?

12. Also, start writing on your 'Your Ecstatic Health Journal'. This is a bonus that you can access at www. LoveyourGutbook.com Think about how your body feels and how you are feeling emotionally at the end of each day, and then write this down in 'Your Ecstatic Health Journal'.

    Again, this might be a little difficult at first, but it will become easier as you get into the habit. Think about and record your energy levels each day. Record your energy levels on a scale of between 1 and 10 out of 10 each day. Look to see if there are connections between your energy levels and certain foods that you eat.

    'Your Ecstatic Health Journal' will make for a fabulous read when you get to the end of the 90 days. It will constitute a record of the success that you have achieved. Thus, I would encourage you at the end to take the time to sit down and read it and really take on board your success and celebrate that with yourself.

Week 2.

1. Continue as in Week 1, but try to reduce more of the sugar you are consuming during the week.

2. After you have eaten a particular food such as bread or cakes and biscuits, start to listen to your body, and think about how your body feels. What are you noticing?

Now the entire situation of reducing sugar in your diet might be setting off some stressful thoughts, so I have provided some tips below on how you can help yourself to manage the cravings for sugar.

There will be a need, though, to have some willpower as you embark on this journey. If you haven't already done the exercise in Chapter 1 to create your vision of how you want your life to be, I would encourage you to go back and do that. Then, when you feel that need to eat sugary things or carbohydrates, bring into your mind the vision of the slimmer, healthy, lovelier you as a reminder as to why you are going to do this and going to achieve the result that you want.

Get yourself some support.

I would highly recommend for you to get a friend that you trust on board, who is totally supportive of you. This person can then support you along this journey. It will then be someone you can turn to when you get those cravings or when you feel that you are struggling. Your friend can help you stay on track.

Tips to Help You with Sugar Cravings

- Start the day by putting a 1 tablespoon (15ml) of freshly squeezed lemon juice (unwaxed and organic, preferably) into a cup of warm water. You can also have another cup later in the day, too.

- Alternatively, you can use 1 tablespoon of apple cider vinegar instead of lemon juice.

- I would encourage you to eat little amounts but often with snacks between meals. I highly recommend my Crunchy Munchy Seeds. These are a great alternative to something that you might normally have as a snack as they are very healthful and packed with nutrition. They are also very tasty. You will find the recipe for these in Chapter 6.

- Other things to snack on are nuts—almonds or pecans. These should be raw and not roasted. Coconut chips are great too. You can get these from health food and whole food shops. These items will help to regulate your blood sugar.

Access your Free 'Your Ecstatic Health Journal'
for you to log the physical and emotional changes
that you experience as you go through this journey
at www.loveyourgutbook.com.

CHAPTER 6

Your Ecstatic Health Eating Plan™

'We can change our lives. We can do, have, and be exactly what we wish'.

—*Tony Robbins*

Basic Principles

THE BASIC PRINCIPLE OF YOUR Ecstatic Health Eating Plan is to address your gut health and get it into an authentically healthy condition. We address this by taking out from your eating plan the types of foods that are having a negative effect on your gut health and the alkalinity of your body. We then focus on the types of foods that support a healthy body and immune system.

If you truly want to accomplish a health transformation and achieve weight loss, you really do have to follow the process as it has been set out in this book.

Along with not eating sugar, gluten, yeast, and dairy products from cows' milk, Your Ecstatic Health Eating Plan also uses the principle of not eating protein together with carbohydrates. These two types of foods need different enzymes and a different environment in the gut to be both properly digested. Eating both of these types of foods together means that neither get properly digested. This combination will then have a negative effect, for the food will not pass through your system effectively and start to break down.

I can assure that you will not be starving or hungry. You will just be putting lovely, natural, tasty, healthful, and nutritious foods into your body, and your body is going to thank you for it. You will be amazed at how well you start to feel in a quite a short time.

Getting Started

During the first two weeks of starting this process you are going to do these things:

1. Start to reduce the foods that you won't be eating when you go forward as explained in Chapter 5.

2. Review and clear your cupboards and fridge of foods that you will not be eating and eliminate foods that are old and no longer fresh as explained in Chapter 5.

3. Get everything ready by buying the foods, vitamins, and supplements that you will need as part of Your Ecstatic Health Eating Plan.

Detox Symptoms

When you start this new lifestyle eating plan, you will be embarking on a process that will start to cleanse your body. As a result, you will probably get symptoms of your body detoxifying.

These are some of the things you may experience:

- Headaches

- Loss of appetite

- Fatigue

- Spots erupting

- Fever

- Nausea

The main reason for starting the programme with a 2-week gentle ease-in to your new way of eating is to limit these detoxification symptoms as much as possible. I know that some of you may find managing any detox symptoms a bit of a challenge, especially as it will come at the beginning of your body's transformation process. But do stick with it, for your body will feel fantastic at the end of the 90 days. You will be very pleased that you persevered. Maintain the end result that you want by visualising what you will look and feel like at the end of the 90 days. It is all going to be worth it, and the symptoms will only last for a few days.

At the end, you will feel amazing, and your body will truly thank you for it.

To help with these symptoms, you should do the following:

- Drink lots of filtered or mineral water to flush the toxins out of your body. You should be drinking about 8 pints per day. The more you can drink, the quicker the symptoms will disappear.

- Take 6 teaspoons of olive oil.

- Dry skin brush before you shower every morning.

- Go for a walk outside and get some fresh air.

- Take 1 tablespoon of linseeds soaked in water for a couple of hours. Swallow these with plenty of water before breakfast.

- Get plenty of rest and relaxation.

Tracking Your Progress

You can weigh and measure yourself when you start the programme, but then a key rule is not to do that again until you have completed the 90 days. I would start the programme on a Monday. That will make it easier for you to keep track of which week you are on. I want you to notice your bodily changes as they occur. It serves no purpose to be constantly weighing since that just causes stress and tension and makes you focus on the negative. There is no point to this at all.

I would encourage you to get someone to take a photo of you at the start of this journey and then to take one at the end so that you can truly see your achievement. It is a strange thing, but when we look in the mirror at ourselves, we don't seem to see the changes because they are happening slowly over a period of time. Do you find that to be true? People will make comments about the changes they see and compliment you, but it is likely you will not notice them as much as they do. So listen to them and not to yourself because they are seeing correctly and you are not.

I will be talking about the whole subject of compliments in Chapter 9.

You can access the 'Your Ecstatic Health Body Profile Chart' at www.loveyourgutbook.com to log your starting and finishing weight and body measurements.

My recommendation is not to start Your Ecstatic Health Eating Plan if you are about to go on holiday. That might make it a little challenging at first, and it would be better to ensure that you have a totally relaxing holiday and then come back fresh and ready to start the process for the 90 days. Whilst I say this programme is for the next 90 days, I know that you will want to continue to eat in this way after the 90 days is over. The reason for me saying that is that you are going to be feeling so terrific that it won't even enter into your head to go back to eating the way you are now.

Nevertheless, I do know that you won't believe me right now. Of course, most of my clients don't. But they do come back to me at the end saying, 'You know when I said at the beginning that I could go back to eating the way I used to after the 90 days, and you said I wouldn't want to. Well you were absolutely right. I feel so great, why would I want to go back to my old way of eating?"

If you have a partner and feel that you may have to cook different food for yourself because your partner does not want to eat like you, then you may be interested to read this testimonial from one of my clients. This is a comment from a client whose partner joined her on Your Ecstatic Health Eating Plan:

> 'Also, my partner, who is a type 2 diabetic, has had some incredible results by just eating the same as me. He says the food is tasty and delicious and doesn't really want to go back to the way we ate before. Our energy levels have soared, and we both feel fantastic'.
> —Caroline, Nottingham

I have provided a list below of all the things that you are going to need to follow Your Ecstatic Health Eating Plan.

Shopping List

For Yourself

Buy a natural bristle brush for dry skin brushing. This can be obtained from most health food stores. Make sure you get a medium strength as a hard one will not be good for when you start skin brushing.

Also, buy a small notebook. If you are a woman, I would recommend that you get a really nice, pretty, feminine one for yourself.

Vitamins/Minerals and Supplements

- Natural organic multivitamin and minerals
- High quality probiotic
- L-Glutamine – This works on healing the gut.
- Milk thistle – This supports the liver through any detox.

You will need both the caprylic acid and the grapefruit seed extract to start Week 6 of the programme. These are natural anti-fungals.

- Grapefruit seed extract
- Caprylic acid 500mg

Regarding the vitamins and supplements, I recommend buying high quality, organic, naturally produced products. It is also important to check that they are free from gluten, soy, wheat, lactose, added sugar, salt, yeast and preservatives. You will need these for the full 90 days of the programme. I would also recommend that you keep taking the multivitamins and minerals and the probiotic on an ongoing basis and keep taking caprylic acid and grapefruit seed extract on alternate weeks for a further 3 months after you have completed the first 90 days. It will be beneficial to not to take the same pro-biotic on a continuous basis, but to swap after a month or so with a different one.

Taking Vitamins and Supplements

You should start taking the following from Week 1:

- Multivitamin and mineral supplement
- Milk thistle
- L-Glutamine
- Probiotic

Then you will be on a rotation of caprylic acid and grapefruit seed extract on a weekly basis from Week 6. I recommend that you write down on your weekly journal sheet, which supplement you are taking for that week to avoid any confusion.

Important:

Follow the instructions provided by the manufacturers on the bottles for the dosage needed for vitamins and supplements.

For the Kitchen

A water filter

The preferable choice is an alkaline water filter jug and filters, but other ones are fine too. Ensure that you buy 3 spare filters although they do tend to last around 1 month to 6 weeks. You don't want to run out!

Stainless steel steamer

Wok for quick cooking and stir frying

Hard brush for scrubbing organic vegetables

You'll need glass containers, preferably for storing food to take to work or when travelling or just for storing in the fridge, but plastic ones are acceptable. Screw-top, sealed glass storage jars or rubber-sealed, spring-top jars are magnificent for storing nuts and seeds and spices and other loose items such as brown rice flakes, quinoa, etc. And they are low cost also.

Food processor and/or liquidiser. A handheld blender is useful for making soups.

A set of measuring cups

Pressure cooker – This is very useful for cooking brown rice quickly but not essential if you don't already have one.

Ingredients

This is meant as a list to get started with some of the basic ingredients you will need. It is not an exhaustive list of all you will need whilst on the programme. You may also already have some of the things listed. So I suggest you put a tick against those items that you don't have or need to replace if yours are old or out of date.

Cold-pressed extra virgin olive oil

Organic apple cider vinegar

Organic Virgin Coconut Oil

Yeast free vegetable stock. These are available from good health stores.

Sea salt or pink Himalayan salt

Black pepper

Organic brown rice flakes

Organic quinoa flakes

Organic buckwheat flakes

Organic brown rice

Organic brown rice pasta

Buckwheat groats/chips – This is not a grain or a form of wheat. It is a useful replacement for grains.

Coconut milk or coconut block

Organic sunflower seeds

Organic sesame seeds that are not hulled

Organic pumpkin seeds

Organic seaweed sprinkle

Braggs liquid aminos – This is available from your local health food shop or online

Raw tahini

Raw organic garlic

Maca powder – This can be purchased from health shops or online.

Lucuma powder – This can be purchased from health shops or online.

Cinnamon

Curry powder

Cumin powder

Coriander powder

Basil

Oregano

Thyme

Chilli powder

Cornflour

Nutmeg

Curry paste – choose one that has the hotness you prefer.

Herbal teas – peppermint, camomile, three ginger, rooibos—green or normal. You can have a green rooibos tea, which is a good alternative if you normally like to drink green tea as this one is caffeine free.

Almond milk – Please make sure that it is unsweetened. It is really important to ensure that it doesn't have sugar in it as many brands do. You will find that the ones on the refrigerated shelves in supermarkets do contain sugar. Also avoid the ones that have carrageenan gum as well. This is not good for your health. I encourage you to check the ingredients before purchasing.

Organic almonds – raw not roasted. Along with eating

these as a snack, you will process them in a food processor to make your own ground almonds.

Organic pecan nuts – raw not roasted

Organic linseeds/flaxseeds – These can be called either linseeds or flaxseeds, but they are the same thing. Golden would be my preference, but it doesn't matter whether you choose the golden or the brown variety.

Root ginger

Soft goats cheese – no rind

Live goat's yoghurt or coconut yoghurt – These are available in most supermarkets and health shops.

Gluten-free oatcakes – These are available from super-markets or wholefood/health shops.

Rice cakes - plain

Organic/free-range eggs

Organic pulses – lentils, butterbeans, chickpeas, or red kidney beans; Tinned or carton versions can be used for quickness. I'd use the ones in cartons in preference to those in tins.

Cans of tuna and sardines

Goat's butter

Goat's milk – You don't need to use goat's milk if you don't like it. It is just there as an option. You can just use almond milk instead.

Whilst I recommend that you buy organic products, they are not essential. I am aware that this may not be possible due to budget restrictions, but try and buy as much organic as you can.

Your Ecstatic Health Eating Plan

In order to get you started, here are some examples of recipes for food that you will be eating over the next 90 days. In fact, I know that at the end of the 90 days, you will continue to eat this way because you are going to feel so remarkable .

Breakfast Ideas and Options:

Brown Rice Porridge

Serves 1

Ingredients:

½ cup brown rice flakes

1 cup filtered water

1 cup of unsweetened almond milk

2 dspn of flax/linseeds

1 dspn of sesame seeds

1 dspn of desiccated coconut

1 tsp of cinnamon

1 tsp of maca

Place the ½ cup of brown rice flakes into a saucepan with the water and almond milk. Bring to a boil and then simmer for 10 minutes.

In the meantime, place all the other ingredients into a serving bowl. Then add the cooked brown rice flakes to your ingredients and stir everything until fully mixed. If this makes for too thick a consistency, add more almond milk and mix until you reach the desired quality.

You can create variety in the porridge by using buckwheat flakes or quinoa flakes instead of brown rice flakes.

Chia Seed Breakfast Delight

Serves 1

This is a very quick and easy breakfast that you make the night before. It is also highly portable if you make it in a glass container with a lid. You can then take it with you.

Ingredients:

   1 cup of unsweetened almond milk

   3 tbsp of organic chia seeds

   2 tbsp of organic desiccated coconut

   1 tbsp of organic cocoa nibs

   1 tsp of lucuma powder

   1 dspn ground almonds

All of these items can be bought from good health food shops either in store on online. Check that your almond milk is unsweetened as quite a lot of them are sweetened in some way.

You can make your own ground almonds by putting raw whole almonds into a food processor and blitzing/grinding them until they are reasonably fine.

You will need a small mixing bowl in which you add all of the ingredients one by one. A 1pt bowl will be fine. First add the almond milk and then add all the other ingredients.

When everything is added into the mixing bowl, give it all a really good stir round. If you are looking to take this with you somewhere in the morning—to eat at work, for example—then make it in a glass container that has a lid.

Cover the bowl and place in the fridge overnight. In the morning it will have turned into a thick consistency.

Middle Eastern Eggs

Serves 2

Ingredients:

1 tin of chopped tomatoes

1 tsp cumin powder

1 tsp coriander powder

4 free range eggs

1 onion chopped

1 clove garlic chopped

1 dspn of coconut oil

Sea salt to taste

Ground pepper to taste

In a medium-sized frying pan, ideally with a lid, add the coconut oil and melt. Then add the chopped onion and chopped garlic and fry until soft and golden.

Add the tinned tomatoes to the fried onion and garlic in the frying pan and cook for 15 minutes. Then make four holes in the tomato mixture and crack an egg into each of the 4 spaces.

Place a lid over the frying pan and simmer on low heat until the eggs are of the consistency that you prefer. If you like your egg soft, then cook for 5 minutes. If you like the egg hard, then leave for a further 5 minutes.

Serve 2 eggs per person with the tomato mixture.

Soaked Muesli

Serves 2

Ingredients:

¼ cup of brown rice flakes

¼ cup of buckwheat flakes

2 cups of unsweetened almond milk

You can mix together any combination of two types of these items listed according to what you like and for variety: ¼ cup of gluten-free oats or quinoa or millet flakes. So you could have brown rice flakes and gluten free oats, buckwheat flakes and quinoa flakes, or brown rice flakes and millet flakes. The choice is yours.

Add all the ingredients to a bowl and leave overnight to soak. In the morning add some linseeds, sunflower seeds, desiccated coconut and sesame seeds. Stir, and if necessary to get to the right consistency, add extra unsweetened almond milk.

Other Ideas for Breakfast Options:

Omelette with steamed spinach

Tomato scrambled egg

Poached egg on rice cake or gluten-free oat cake

Plain scrambled egg

Lunch Ideas and Options:

Soups with salads are a great idea because they are so easily portable. So you can make them at home and then take them into work with you. Soups alone are great too because they can be made very quickly from scratch with vegetables, and you can also freeze portions in your freezer and then heat them up for a quick lunch.

You also have the opportunity to get creative and make up your own combinations using different vegetable combinations with herbs and spices.

Here are some of my favourites:

Chick Pea Red Pepper Soup

Serves 2

Ingredients:

1 tin of chickpeas drained and rinsed in a sieve until water runs clear

1 tsp of coconut oil

1 medium onion

1 clove of garlic, finely chopped

1 large red pepper, deseeded and chopped into small pieces

1 teaspoon of cumin powder

300ml or ½pt yeast free vegetable stock – add 1 stock cube to ½ pt/300ml of boiled water

Salt and pepper to taste

Put the coconut oil into a pan, and then add the chopped onion and garlic and fry until translucent.

Add the stock to the pan, and then add the red pepper and the chickpeas and the cumin powder. Bring to the boil, and then simmer for 20 minutes.

Pour into a blender or use a handheld blender and blend until smooth. Serve.

Mixed Winter Vegetable Soup

Serves 2

Reserve one portion and freeze for use next week.

1 leek, washed and chopped into small pieces

2 carrots peeled and chopped into small pieces

2 sticks of celery washed and chopped into small pieces

1 medium onion, sliced and chopped finely

1 potato peeled and chopped into small cubes

500ml of stock made with boiled water and 1 yeast-free stock cube

½ tsp of thyme

1 tbsp Extra Virgin olive oil

Salt and pepper to taste

Place the olive oil in a saucepan, and fry the onion until translucent. Then add all the other vegetables to the pan.

Pour on the vegetable stock, and add the thyme and salt and pepper to taste. Simmer for around 15-20 minutes until all the vegetables are cooked. Then blend until smooth. Serve.

Green Vegetable Soup
Serves 2

Ingredients:

1 medium onion, chopped

1 large courgette, washed and sliced

1 handful of washed watercress

2 sticks of celery, washed and sliced thickly

1 tsp of coconut oil

250 gms of French beans washed and chopped into small pieces

¼ tsp nutmeg

½ tsp thyme

½ tsp basil

1 cup of filtered water

1 yeast-free vegetable stock cube

Heat the coconut oil in a saucepan, and add the onion and fry until soft and translucent.

Add the courgette, watercress, celery and beans to the pan with the water, stock cube, nutmeg, thyme and basil.

Bring to the boil and then simmer for 20 minutes until the vegetables are cooked. Using a blender, blend the soup until smooth. Serve.

Here are some other options for lunch:

Salad "Sort of Nicoise"

Serves 1

Ingredients:

  2 free-range eggs, hard boiled

  Mixed salad leaves, spinach, rocket, lettuce

  6 cherry or small plum tomatoes – halved

  2" piece of cucumber sliced

  ½ a ripe avocado chopped into small pieces

Place 2 eggs in a pan of cold water and bring to the boil. Then simmer for 10 minutes.

Once cooked, pour off the hot water and place the eggs into cold water.

Vinaigrette

  2 dspn Extra Virgin olive oil

  1 dspn apple cider vinegar

  ½ small clove of garlic – optional

  Sea salt and ground black pepper to taste

Place the olive oil and vinegar in a serving bowl, add the chopped garlic, and add salt and pepper to taste. Mix together.

To Finish:

Then add the salad leaves, cucumber, tomatoes, and avocado to the vinaigrette and mix well.

Peel and quarter the hard boiled eggs, and place on top of the salad.

Hummus and Crudités

You'll need a mesh strainer or colander, food processor, silicone spatula, and measuring cups and spoons.

This will make about 1½ cups or enough for 4 to 6 snack portions. It can be stored in an airtight container in the fridge for 1 week.

Ingredients:

One 15-ounce can (425 grams) chickpeas

¼ cup (59 ml) fresh lemon juice, about 1 large lemon

¼ cup (59 ml) tahini

Half of a large garlic clove, minced

2 tablespoons olive oil, plus more for serving

½ to 1 tsp sea salt, depending on taste

½ tsp ground cumin

2 to 3 tbsp water

Dash of ground paprika for serving

Crudités

1 stick of organic celery – washed and chopped into 3" pieces

3" piece of organic cucumber – cut into quarters as sticks

½ of an organic red pepper – stalk and seeds removed, then sliced into ½" strips

5 cherry or small plum tomatoes

Method

In the bowl of a food processor, combine tahini and lemon juice. Process for 1 minute. Scrape sides and bottom of bowl, then turn on and process for 30 seconds. This extra time helps 'whip' or 'cream' the tahini, making smooth and creamy hummus possible.

Add the olive oil, minced garlic, cumin, and salt to the whipped tahini and lemon juice mixture. Process for 30 seconds, scrape the sides and bottom of bowl. Then process for another 30 seconds.

Open the can of chickpeas, drain liquid, and then rinse well with water. Add half of the chickpeas to the food processor then process for 1 minute. Scrape sides and bottom of bowl, add remaining chickpeas, and process for 1 to 2 minutes or until thick and quite smooth.

To create the right consistency:

It is most likely that the hummus will be too thick or still have tiny bits of chickpea. To fix this, with the food processor turned on, slowly add 2 to 3 tablespoons of water until the consistency is perfect.

To serve, scrape the hummus into a bowl, and then drizzle about 1 tablespoon of olive oil over the top, and sprinkle with paprika.

Place the crudités on a plate, and place a portion of hummus in the centre. Then dip the crudités into the hummus, and enjoy. It's great eating food with your hands, but make sure you have washed them first!

71

Guacamole with Gluten Free Oatcakes

Serves 2

Ingredients

2 ripe avocados, peeled, stone removed, and mashed

1 large tomato, finely chopped

1 small onion, chopped finely

½ tsp minced garlic

Juice of 1 lime

½ teaspoon sea salt

2 tbsp chopped fresh coriander

Pinch of ground cayenne pepper

Combine all the ingredients, and mix thoroughly. Serve with gluten-free oatcakes, or you could—as an alternative—use crudités to dip in. For example, sticks of celery, carrot, and cucumber.

Another quick and easy option, particularly if you have roast meat left over on a Sunday, is to serve that cold with a mixed salad.

Spanish Omelette with Salad

Serves 2

Ingredients

For the Omelette

6 free-range eggs

1 dspn of olive oil

2 chopped small courgettes

1 chopped medium onion

1 red pepper de-seeded and chopped into small pieces

Sea salt and ground black pepper to taste

For the Salad

Mixed salad leaves, spinach, rocket, lettuce,

2 dspn extra virgin olive oil

1 dspn apple cider vinegar

1 small clove of garlic – optional

1 tsp dried oregano

Sea salt and ground black pepper to taste

Vinaigrette

Place the olive oil and vinegar in a serving bowl, add the chopped garlic, and add salt and pepper to taste. Mix together.

Add the salad leaves and mix thoroughly.

Prepare the Omelette

Crack the eggs into a small bowl, and beat until white and yolk are well mixed. Add a splodge (dab) of almond milk. Add salt and pepper to taste.

Heat the olive oil in the frying pan, and then add the onion and red pepper and fry gently on a low heat until soft. Add the sliced courgette, and fry for 10 minutes. When the courgettes are soft and golden brown, sprinkle the oregano over them. Then pour in the beaten egg mixture, and cook gently for 10-15 minutes until the egg has gone solid.

Next, place the pan under a grill for a couple of minutes or until golden brown. Cut the omelette into quarters, and serve with the green salad.

If you are at home during the day, you may want to choose to have the larger meal for your dinner menu at lunch time and then have lunch options in the evening. The choice is yours to fit into your lifestyle.

Dinner Ideas and Options:

Vegetable Chilli

Ingredients:

1 dspn of organic coconut oil

1 large onion, finely chopped

2 cloves of garlic sliced

2 medium sized courgettes – sliced and quartered

1 red pepper – chopped

2 leeks trimmed and chopped into ½ inch slices

1 can or carton of organic red kidney beans – strained and washed in a sieve until the water runs clear

1 tin of canned, organic, chopped tomatoes

½ to 1 tsp of chilli powder – depending on how hot you like it and how hot your chilli powder is; suggest erring on the side of caution if you don't know

1 yeast-free vegetable stock cube

¼ cup of boiled water

Salt and pepper to taste

Melt the coconut oil in a medium-sized saucepan. Fry the chopped onion and garlic in the oil until soft and translucent.

Add the chopped courgette, red pepper, leeks, and the can of red kidney beans. Then add the chopped tomatoes.

Dissolve the stock cube in the ¼ cup of boiled water, and then add to the pan with the vegetables together with the chilli powder.

Add salt and pepper taste.

Bring to the boil, and then simmer for 20 minutes. Then serve.

Quick-and-Easy Vegetable Stir Fry
Serves 4

Ingredients

3 cloves of garlic

2.5 cm/1" piece of root ginger

125 gm/4.5 oz of carrots sliced and then quartered

125 gm/4.5 oz of mange tout, trimmed

125 gm/4.5 oz of green beans sliced

1 yellow pepper, deseeded and chopped

1 red pepper, deseeded and chopped

1 dspn virgin coconut oil

2 tbsp water

450 gm/1lb broccoli, cut up into small florets

1 tbsp Bragg Liquid Aminos

4 spring onions

Salt and pepper to taste

Peel and finely chop the garlic, and peel and grate the ginger.

Heat the oil in a wok, then add the garlic and ginger and stir-fry for 1 minute. Add the broccoli, peppers and carrots. Stir-fry for 5 minutes.

Add the water, mange tout, and green beans to the wok, and cook for a further 5 minutes. Now stir in the Bragg Liquid Aminos.

Trim and finely chop the spring onions and sprinkle over. Season, give one last stir, and serve immediately.

Buckwheat and Lemon-Crusted Mackerel
Serves 2

Ingredients:

2 tbsp buckwheat flakes

Grated rind of 1 unwaxed lemon

2 tbsp sea vegetable seasoning

220 gm/8 oz fresh mackerel fillets

Mix all the ingredients together, except the fish, and put on a plate. Press the fish into the mixture so that the fillet surface is covered. Heat the grill to its highest setting. Oil the grill grid, and arrange the fillets on the grid.

Grill for 4 minutes on high. Then turn the grill down to

medium. Turn the fish, and continue cooking for another 4-5 minutes. Turn off the grill, and leave the fish to rest for a couple of minutes before serving.

Serve with a mixed salad.

Middle Eastern Roast Vegetables

Serves 4

Ingredients:

1 aubergine cut into 2 cm cubes

2 red onions, quartered

2 cloves garlic, crushed and chopped

1 celeriac (fist size) peeled, cubed, and plunged into cold water with a splash of cider vinegar to stop it from going brown

3 carrots, peeled and cut into chunks

2 green peppers, deseeded, membrane-removed, and sliced in to 2cm strips

300 gms fresh ripe tomatoes, chopped

1 tin of chick peas, rinsed and drained

1 tsp coriander powder

1 tsp cumin powder

1 cup coriander leaves, roughly chopped.

200 ml Extra Virgin olive oil

Pre-heat the oven to 220°C/425°F/Gas Mark 7

In a bowl, mix the aubergine, onion, garlic, celeriac, peppers, carrots, spices, seasoning, and the olive oil. Then spread out evenly in on a large baking tray, and place in the oven. Cook for 10 minutes, then gently turn the vegetables, and roast for a further 20 minutes, turning occasionally so they colour evenly.

Remove from the oven, and incorporate the tomatoes and the chick peas. Then return to the oven for a further 10 minutes. Remove from the oven again, add the chopped coriander, and serve.

Vegetable Buckwheat Risotto

Serves 4

Ingredients:

175 gms/6 oz buckwheat grains, rinsed

1 litre/1¾ pints yeast-free vegetable stock

2 tbsp olive oil

2 tbsp chopped fresh parsley

2 medium onions finely chopped

1 clove garlic finely chopped

225 gm/8 oz of broccoli, divided into florets and with slices of stalk

225 gm/8 oz carrots, grated

1 red pepper, deseeded, and sliced and chopped into small pieces

Cook the buckwheat in the stock. Bring to the boil, and then simmer for 30 minutes. After 20 minutes, add the broccoli and the carrots, and continue cooking. Drain the buckwheat.

Heat the olive oil, and gently fry the onions and the garlic until translucent.

Stir in the buckwheat and vegetables and chopped parsley. Serve with your favourite green vegetable.

Pancake Cottage Pie
Serves 3

Pancake Batter

   115 gms of buckwheat flour

   1 egg, beaten

   285 ml/ ½ pt of unsweetened almond milk

Put the flour into a bowl, and add the egg. Beat together, and then slowly add the almond milk while beating continuously. Finish by whisking the batter, and then leave to stand.

   1 tsp of coconut oil

   1 medium onion, chopped

   1 lb of minced beef

   1 carrot, peeled and sliced

   250 ml yeast-free vegetable stock made with 1 stock cube.

Put the coconut oil into a saucepan. Fry the onion until translucent. Add the mince until it is all brown, and keep moving it to ensure there are no clumps. Add the sliced carrot, and then add the stock. Bring to the boil, and then simmer for 25 minutes.

Heat the oven to 180°C/350°F/Gas Mark 4

To Cook the Pancakes

Use ½ tsp of olive oil to grease the pan for each pancake made. Choose a pan that has a similar diameter to the ovenproof dish you will use for the mince.

You just want a light thin covering of oil on the surface of the pan. Make sure that the pan and oil are very hot before starting to cook a pancake. Add just enough of the batter to thinly spread round the pan. Then leave to cook until the mixture solidifies. You will see little holes appearing. At this point, flip over the pancake and cook on the other side for a couple of minutes. Place the cooked pancakes onto a plate. Go through this process until you have used all the batter.

Using an ovenproof, round deep dish, place one pancake in the bottom, and then add a layer of mince. Then add another pancake, and then mince, until you have used 4 pancakes and all the mince. You finish with a pancake on the top. If there are pancakes left over, you can freeze these to use next week, and fill them with stir fried vegetables.

Place the dish of mince and pancakes into the oven for 15 minutes.

Serve with steamed green beans.

Summary of Eating Principles

In general, you can eat cooked fresh meat or fish grilled or roasted and served with lots of vegetables (not potatoes) or a green or mixed salad. However, I would recommend only eating meat/fish 2 to 3 times per week. It is best also to have vegetarian dishes made with a good mix of vegetables including different types of beans and pulses. It is also better to switch the balance to eating more vegetables and less meat. The amount of food you will want to consume will naturally decrease over the weeks.

If you need help, and also for ease, you can access sample menus and further recipes at www.loveyourgutbook.com.

Handy Time-Saving Tip

You can double up on the quantities of the cooked recipes you make and eat one portion and freeze the other. That way, when you have moments when you are short of time, you will be sure to still be eating according to Your Ecstatic Health Eating Plan™

Snacks

If you feel that you need a snack in the mid-morning or mid-afternoon, then pour yourself a big glass of water to drink first. It might be that you are thirsty rather than hungry. If after 20 minutes of drinking the water, you are still feeling hungry, then snack on a few almond or pecan nuts, coconut chips, or Crunchy Munchy Seeds. The recipe for these is below:

Crunchy Munchy Seeds: A Highly Nutritious and Tasty Snack

Ingredients:

1 cup of organic sunflower seeds

1 cup of organic pumpkin seeds

½ cup of organic sesame seeds

2 dspn of Bragg Liquid Aminos (This is an unfermented soy sauce similar to tamari.)

Preheat the oven to 150°C/300°F/Gas Mark 2

Place the sunflower and pumpkin seeds onto a large oven-baking tray and roast in the oven for 15 minutes. Be aware that if you have a fan-assisted oven, these may take less time. Remove from the oven, and add the sesame seeds. Give them a stir round with a spoon. Then place back into the oven for a further 5 minutes.

Remove from the oven, and sprinkle over the Bragg Aminos. Give them a good stir, and turn over the seeds several times. Return to the oven for a further 5 minutes. Remove from the oven, and leave to cool before storing in a screw-top glass jar.

I recommend using airtight preserving jars. These screw-top jars are available in different sizes from kitchen/hardware stores or kitchen departments in department stores. Storing the seeds in smaller jars means that you can have some on your desk at work or take them away with you or keep some in the car. This way you won't need to resort to eating things you shouldn't be eating.

To be totally clear about each of the things that you need to be taking in terms of vitamins and supplements, as well as eating, you can access a bonus 'Your Ecstatic Health Daily Reminder Sheet for Weeks 1-5 and for Weeks 1- 6' at www. loveyourgutbook.com.

You can get lots of tips on how to cope with eating out and travelling in the next chapter.

You can access your free bonus recipe book, some example menus, the 'Your Ecstatic Health Body Profile Chart', and the Daily Reminder sheets at www.loveyourgutbook. com.

CHAPTER 7

How To Deal With Eating Out

*'A man too busy to take care of his health is like a
mechanic too busy to take care of his tools'.*
—*Spanish Proverb*

When you are eating differently from the way you used to, one
of the key problems is how to deal with this when eating out,
when you are travelling or are on holiday. This can be a little
daunting, and obviously, you don't want to undo the great work
that you have already done by going back and eating the foods
that don't serve your body or your health.

So I am going to provide you with some key tips to make the process of staying on track with eating in this new way dead simple.

These are the key situations where you will be faced with having
to make the right food choices:

1. Going to work
2. Early morning starts

3. Networking events
4. Travelling
5. Holidays
6. Eating out in restaurants
7. Dinner parties

Whilst you are on this body and health transformational journey, and certainly in the early stages, I would recommend that you avoid eating out and avoid succumbing to the temptation of getting a take-away. The reason for this is that you and your body need time to adjust, and eating out may put additional pressures on you that won't help you at this time.

On the other hand, I am certainly not advocating that you give up social contact because this is very important to your health and wellbeing.

The key to successful eating out of your home is really in the planning. Planning ahead and making sure you have things to take with you, checking the menu in advance for a restaurant or an event venue, and submitting your dietary requirements in advance to event organisers will mean the difference between a calm, easy experience and a stressful one. It could also mean the difference between being hungry and well satisfied.

1. Going to Work

If you are used to just grabbing a sandwich and some crisps and coffee or a coke or doing something similar for lunch, then this whole routine will need to change. The key thing will be thinking ahead and planning what you are going to have for your lunch and what snacks you might want to keep at work.

This may seem like a bit of a chore at first, but once you get into the habit, it will soon become second nature to you. Change your thoughts to one of How I am going to nourish my body with good food, which is going to make me feel more healthy and more energetic? It is really just about changing your mindset.

The ideal scenario would be for you to prepare a lunch at home to take into work each day, but I am well aware that this isn't always possible. Even so, this plan will save you money. So how about putting the money that you would normally spend on coffees and lunch and snacks at work each day into a tin or piggy bank? Then you could use this money to buy yourself a new outfit to celebrate your success in losing weight and feeling so much healthier. That would be a great reward to yourself for honouring your body and your health. It would also be a good thing to focus on when you feel like things are a little difficult.

You will soon reap the rewards of eating this way, and you will notice that you don't have energy dips after lunch, so your productivity is going to be so much better at work in the afternoon.

Also, if you have typically avoided having breakfast or just grabbed something and a coffee as you were on your way to work, you are also going to notice how more productive and effective you are in the morning at work too. A good healthful breakfast is really important to ensure that you balance your energy levels in the morning. Your brain cannot work effectively without good food and enough fluid.

Here are some ideas for foods that you can prepare for lunch:

i. Mixed Salad

A mixed salad of green leaves, tomatoes, and cucumber, with your own homemade vinaigrette dressing. You could add some soft goat's cheese or some grilled or roasted chicken or some grilled fish or two hard boiled eggs to the salad. You could also add cooked green beans, avocado, oven-roasted courgette, or aubergine. There are lots of options you can put together to create variety. Put this into a glass fridge box and its ready to go.

ii. Fresh Vegetable Soup

Prepare some fresh vegetable soup the night before. You can then heat this up in the morning, put it into a vacuum flask, and take it to work and have it with 2 gluten free oatcakes or a rice cake.

Or you can make soup in bulk on the weekend, when you have more time, and then freeze it into meal-size portions. This will make this whole process very easy.

iii. Hummus with Vegetable Crudités

Prepare some homemade hummus, and then cut up some celery, carrot, cucumber, and red pepper into strips. These can then be put into a glass fridge box and kept in the fridge overnight, ready to take in the morning.

If you have to buy a lunch out, then look for green salad. Avoid all salads with pasta, noodles, couscous, or croutons as these all contain gluten. A salad with rice would be satisfactory. If you are looking to have soup, then you will need to check that the soup is dairy, sugar, yeast, and gluten free.

Snacks

i. Crunchy Munchy Seeds

Healthy snacks that you can take to work are my Crunchy Munchy Seeds. These can be prepared in bulk at the weekend. They only take 20 minutes to make and are so very easy, very tasty, and nutritious. Store them in small glass airtight jars, and you can then take a jar into work to keep on your desk. (See Recipe on Page 81.)

ii. Raw Almonds or Pecan Nuts

Keep a mix of raw almonds and pecan nuts in a small glass fridge box or glass jar in your desk for those moments when you feel peckish, or take them into meetings if you get caught and are late having lunch.

iii. Gluten Free Oat Cakes

iv. Rice Cakes

2. Early Morning Starts

If you have an early morning start, and you feel that you cannot make time to prepare a breakfast that morning, then there are a couple of options that you can prepare the night before. You can then put these in the fridge the night before so they will be ready to eat in the morning.

- Chia Seed Delight Breakfast
- Soaked Muesli

See the breakfast recipe section on pages 60-63.

3. Networking Events

If you go to breakfast networking events, then there are a few options for this scenario in preferred order:

i. Eat one of the options above that you will have prepared the night before you leave.

ii. Contact the organisers and specify your requirements for breakfast in advance.

iii. If it is a cooked English breakfast, then just have fried egg with tomato.

iv. I recommend that you take your own herbal tea bags with you and request hot water, if it is not provided.

If it is a networking lunch, then provide the organisers with your dietary requirements in advance of the event so that they can prepare a meal that works for you. Today, venues are used to providing for people with dietary requirements, so there is no need to feel awkward or uncomfortable about it. Generally, the organiser of the event will typically ask you if you have any special dietary requirements anyway.

You can buy small filtering bottles that you can refill with tap water at the venue because it filters the water as you drink. Most venues tend to only provide tap water to drink, so you should try and avoid this wherever possible. I would advise you check out the different brands and types of water filter bottles because some are not as good as others.

4. Travelling

The key rule when travelling is to make sure that you have some of the snacks listed above with you. It might be that you meet a situation where it is mealtime and you are hungry, but the shops or food facilities to hand do not serve the types of food that you are eating.

In this situation, particularly if you are hungry, it is easy to make the wrong food choice . You want to avoid this situation. So having some snacks with you that you can eat means you can have those rather than choosing something that is not good for you just to satisfy your hunger pangs.

Always carry some snacks (Crunchy Munchy Seeds, gluten free oatcakes, nuts, and your favourite herbal teas) with you.

The basic rule is you will be looking to have plain meat, fish, or eggs with vegetables or salad.

Also, make sure that you take a bottle of filtered or mineral water with you when travelling to ensure that you maintain your hydration levels.

Ideally, take filtered water in a glass or aluminium flask or bottle, if at all possible. Be careful not to leave water in a plastic bottle in your car in the sun or heat. The heat can cause the plasticisers in the bottle to leach into the water, and that is not good for your health.

Also ensure that you take bottles of still mineral water with you. This is a much cheaper option than buying in hotels.

You can buy small filtering bottles that you can refill with tap water at the venue because it filters as you drink. Do your research on these items as some are not as good as others.

5. Holidays

If you are going abroad on holiday, I would recommend that you go prepared by taking the ingredients as an option that you can eat for breakfast with you. It is quite likely that in some countries you may not be able to buy the things you need. Depending on how long you are away, I would take a carton or two of unsweetened almond milk and take with you the ingredients to make at least the soaked muesli or the porridge. For the soaked muesli, you can mix all the ingredients together in a secure plastic container rather than taking several separate containers.

Of course, whilst on holiday, you can have eggs or an omelette for breakfast with green vegetables such as spinach or peppers and tomatoes, but you will need to specify that you don't want them made with butter or milk. Choosing a self-catering holiday option will make the situation a lot simpler and easier for you.

6. Eating Out in Restaurants

There are certain types of cuisine that suit themselves far better to this form of eating than others.

The best ones for you to choose are Middle Eastern, Indian, Thai, Greek, and Italian. The Mediterranean style of eating certainly suits this way of eating better. However, do be aware of tabbouleh and couscous, for these are forms of wheat.

Also, with Indian food you need to check for curries that don't have yoghurt or cream as their ingredients. If you want to have rice with your curry, then I would recommend you go for a vegetable curry so you are not combining meat with carbohydrates. So any tandoori/tikka meals will not be good for you to have since they are marinated in yoghurt.

I would be cautious of open salad bars and raw food, especially in fast-food chains, because of dressings and toppings and oxidation from food lying around for hours.

The types of food you should choose when eating out are things like these:

- Simple fresh fish grilled with vegetables

- Steak with a salad—avoid any sauces

- Omelette with vegetables or a mixed or green salad

- A salad dish with chicken or similar fresh meat or fish

- Roast meat or chicken with vegetables or a mixed or green salad.

I would also recommend avoiding all fast-food chains, motorway service stations, and food at most pubs, unless they are "gastro type" pubs. In many of the chain pub restaurants, the food is brought in already prepared and reheated and is chemically compromised, full of fats and bulked out with wheat. The restaurant staff members don't tend to know what is actually in the food, even if you ask them. So they are not able to prepare food to your specific requirements.

Good independent restaurants, where food is cooked fresh to order, are usually very good and will accommodate your requirements. However, I would recommend that if you haven't eaten at one of these places before that you check in advance by calling to see what you could have from their menu. Smaller family-owned restaurants are usually very willing to work with you. In particular, I have found independent Italian restaurants to be very helpful. Just let them know the things that you cannot eat. Generally, restaurants nowadays are getting used to people having special dietary requirements, and it is not that difficult to get what you want.

When restaurant staff members are helpful, I find that it is a good idea to thank them for their help. There is an increasing number of people with food intolerances these days, and others are making food choices for health reasons. For this reason, if we can encourage restaurants to be more flexible and responsible to special needs often, it will be a major benefit to us all.

Regarding drinks, always choose still mineral water, and avoid drinking tap water. You can have a slice of lemon in the water, but don't take the ice because you will just be adding tap water to your bottle of mineral water.

7. Dinner Parties

My recommendation would be to not accept dinner-party invitations in the early weeks, unless they are from good friends who understand exactly why you are on this health journey. Too often, people can try to derail you from what you are doing, telling you that it won't matter if you go off plan with your eating just for one meal. The may be doing this with good intentions, but they really don't understand the importance of your plan.

If you are invited to a dinner party, and you feel it is important to go, then I would recommend that you tell the hosts that you are on this journey to transform your health and that you would welcome their support. Let them know in advance the things that you cannot eat so that they have plenty of time to take your eating requirements into account. Also, they don't have to make you any special desserts or anything like this because you will tell them that you don't require such accommodations.

The good news is that you will soon become used to the whole process of making the right choices when eating out. It is important that you keep in mind your vision of the healthy, slimmer you and what you want for your life going forward as that will always keep you on track.

Don't be put off if a restaurant staff makes you feel as if you are making their lives difficult. Their job is to serve you in the best way they can; otherwise, the restaurant will lose out on your custom in the long run. So just ask for what you want and ignore them.

You can access your free bonuses at
www.loveyourgutbook.com.

CHAPTER 8

Bringing In The Attitude Of Gratitude

'Happiness cannot be travelled to, owned, earnt, worn, or consumed. Happiness is the spiritual experience of living every minute with love, grace, and gratitude'.
—Denis Waitley

I N THIS CHAPTER, I WANT to share with you some of the amazing strategies that helped me to get out of the place where I was stuck about 4 years ago. I do this because I know that my pointers will help you to genuinely be able to make the changes you would like to make in your life too.

At the beginning of this book, you may remember I shared with you that about 4 years ago I found myself in a black hole. Everything in my life was in a very bad place. I was in a bad place, my health was poor, I was overweight, and for a time, I was even feeling unfulfilled. I really didn't think there was any way that I could change the situation I was in.

However, what I have learnt since then, from working with my clients, is that I am not the only person who has somehow gotten trapped in a place of being stuck. This probably happens to most people at some point in their lives.

You may be quite possibly in that place now, looking for a way to get yourself out of being stuck but feeling totally helpless because you don't think it is possible. I want you to know that I understand totally how you feel. It doesn't feel great, does it? I also want you to know that there is a way to make those changes and to turn your health and your life around. It is all possible, but we do have to take the first step to make those changes. Then it will be amazing how things start to change and opportunities arise that we wouldn't have thought were truly possible before.

The terrible thing it that is so easy to get stuck in that place of negativity. We get bogged down by beliefs that we have inherited from our parents, teachers, and friends. And often, these things tend to hold us back and make things worse. It also means we get trapped in repeating behaviours that do not help us either.

What negative beliefs do you hold about yourself? You see, the negative voice in my mind tells me that I am not good enough, I can't communicate, and I am inferior. What does your negative voice tell you? Is it something in the list below?

I am not good enough.

I am worthless.

I am unwanted.

I am different.

I am flawed.

I am a bad person.

I am not safe.

I am powerless.

I am unlovable.

I can't communicate.

I am inferior.

I am not interesting enough.

I don't matter.

I am plain and dull.

I am always wrong.

I am no good.

I am a mistake.

I am useless.

I am a failure.

I don't deserve anything.

Actually, it doesn't matter which of these quotes your negative voice tells you that you are. Absolutely none of them are true about you or anybody else, for that matter.

Yes, that is right. None of them are true about you!

You are perfect and wonderful just as you are!

The Power of Bringing Gratitude into Your Life

So what is gratitude, and how can it make your life happier?

Gratitude is the feeling of being thankful and showing appreciation for what we have in our lives. Thankfulness and appreciation are a pathway to a life of happiness and wellbeing. When you take time to pause, review your day, and recognise all of the wonderful things in your life, you feel happier. It really helps to focus on the smallest things that you are grateful for every day.

When we take time to appreciate what we have, it keeps us focused on what is already good in our lives. This in turn helps to open up the doorway to allow more goodness to flow into our lives. Who wouldn't want to receive more goodness in their lives?

If this is something that you haven't practised before, it may be that you are finding it a little difficult to believe in its power. In that case, I would encourage you to just trust the process and start practising for yourself. Then notice what changes you start to see in your life and your wellbeing. It will take a little time, so don't expect to see the changes in a couple of days.

What are the changes you can expect to see and feel when you start practising gratitude every day in your life? There are many changes that you will experience.

The Seven Benefits of an Attitude of Gratitude:

1. **You will feel healthier.**

   When you are grateful, you will find that you can live a much better life because your relationship with the world as a whole improves. You then start to feel much better within your body as well. You see, great health is not only about the physical body. It is about mind, body, and spirit. All of these things are interconnected. So when things improve in more than one of these areas, you will see a marked improvement in your health and general wellbeing.

Each area has a beneficial knock-on effect on the other. Ultimately, when you are grateful for your body, you will naturally start to take better care of it.

2. You will feel happier.

When you are more in tune with all that is going well in your life, you start to have a more positive outlook on things. Also, when you focus on the good things that you have in your life, no matter how small, this will have a positive effect on you and will uplift your mood. So start to recognise the things that are good in your life that you may have previously just taken for granted and really feel the joy of having them in your life. Gratitude doesn't have to be for the big things. In fact, the more you focus on all the little things, the better. You might be grateful that you have a car that gets you to work each day because it makes your life easier than having to take public transport. You can also be grateful for the rain because it helps food to grow so that you can eat. And you can be grateful that you have food to eat each day.

3. You will help others to feel better.

Have you ever noticed how it feels when someone doesn't appreciate what you did for them? It makes you not want to help them again in the future because they don't appreciate it, doesn't it? However, when you say, 'Thank you', even if it is for a very small thing, it makes people feel good about themselves. I am sure you have experienced this when people have thanked you for doing something. This then becomes a powerful motivator for them to want to help you again in the future. So take the time to thank people as often as you can.

4. **You will be better equipped to deal with bad times.**

   The reality of life is that there will always be ups and downs. That is just the way it is. The difference comes from how you view the knocks, setbacks, and failures. In the face of setbacks, you can still practice gratitude by not being defeated by them but just seeing them as learning opportunities. You can give thanks to the Universe or God for giving you the opportunity to practice your patience and your strength, for example. You then should focus on the opportunities that failures give you rather than focusing on the negative consequences.

5. **You will become more satisfied with your life.**

   When you focus more on what you do appreciate about your life, you will become more satisfied on a daily basis. So you will be focusing on the good things rather than the bad. This will lead you to not focus on what you are missing in your life but on what blessings you do have. You will then notice that the feeling of gratitude lasts a lot longer and goes a lot deeper than other fleeting sensations you might have.

6. **You will enrich your children's lives.**

   If you can create a home where you practice gratitude, you will find that this rubs off on your children. They will benefit from learning about gratitude, and they will be much happier and calmer children who will feel that life is a good experience for them.

7. **You will see your relationships improve.**

   When you take the time to be more grateful and generous to the people you care most about, you will see your relationships improve significantly. It will make them feel more appreciated and cared for. Then they will start to reflect back those positive feelings to you. So focus on some small things that they have done to help you rather than on the things that they haven't done, and show your appreciation. You will be surprised at how more helpful they will become as a result.

Action Step

Gratitude is definitely something worth practicing and bringing more of into your life. I would encourage you to start doing this today.

Buy yourself a really nice notebook, which can become your 'gratitude book'. Write 5 things that you are grateful for during the day in your notebook every night before you go to sleep. If you are not used to practicing gratitude, then it might be a little difficult at first to come up with 5 things. So start with maybe 3. Then after a couple of weeks, start building this up until you get to 5, and afterwards, increase to 7. Later, when you get really into the swing of it, try and write 10 things you are grateful for every day.

If you have children, it would be wonderful if you could practice thanking them for little things that they have done too. Make sure that you also thank your partner or husband in front of him as well so that he learns the value of gratitude and starts to benefit from the practice as well. At bedtime you could encourage your children to think of two things that they are grateful for in their day.

Free bonuses are available at
www.loveyourgutbook.com.

CHAPTER 9

Cosset, Coddle, And Care – You Are Worth It!

'The first wealth is health'.

—*Ralph Waldo Emerson*

GETTING STARTED ON THE ROAD to good health requires that you start treating yourself with kindness and care. At the heart of this is to start loving yourself for the wonderful person that you truly are. When you start valuing yourself, you will be bringing a number of things into your life that you probably haven't allowed very much before.

You will be doing these things:

   i.   Putting yourself first

  ii.   Asking for help

 iii.   Graciously receiving

 iv.   Regularly exercising.

1. Putting Yourself First

The biggest thing that enabled me to move out from being totally stuck and feeling helpless and unhealthy was making a decision. But the decision was made based only on what I wanted for myself. I put my needs for my life first.

I let go of what effect my decision would have on other people because I couldn't go on living my life for other people. I had to start living my life for me. Life should be fun and enjoyable. That is what we all deserve. It doesn't need to be a difficult struggle.

As a result, I was able to change my life from one of being unhealthy, overweight, unfulfilled, tired, and living to work, to one of enjoyment, fun, total fulfilment, and feeling good about myself.

When you love yourself and look after your own needs first, EVERYTHING in your life benefits. Loving yourself means caring deeply for yourself. It means making your sleep, your nutrition, and your wellbeing a priority in your life. It means making sure that going to the gym, going to a dance class, giving time to a hobby that you love, or just having a relaxing time in a hot bath on a regular basis are non-negotiable.

It might mean cancelling late night plans so that you can get enough sleep or just shutting off the computer or not checking your phone after a certain hour and logging out of social media. It also means scheduling a regular massage on a monthly basis that can't be changed for something else that might get in the way.

This really is about listening to your body and giving it what it needs to feel its best.

All areas of your life will benefit when you start looking after number one and taking care of yourself and your body.

It doesn't matter who we are. We all have the same number of hours in the day. There are only 24 hours for everybody every day. The difference is how we prioritise the way we use those hours. I was once someone who was always on the treadmill, busting a gut to do everything for everybody, feeling stressed all the time, and never having enough hours in the day to get everything done. But I found that when I put myself first, I really started to reap benefits in many different areas of my life.

Here are some of those benefits:

1. **You'll be more productive at work.**

    You will be a much better worker, think more creatively, and execute things faster when you take care of yourself. This means the project that will take your frazzled, overwhelmed mind four hours will take your well-rested, clear head two.

    Ensuring that you get adequate sleep every night will always be worth it. Make your 'me' time a priority, and you will then be able to show up to whatever task you have at hand that day as your best self. Your boss will thank you, and your career will take off much faster if you don't burn yourself out.

2. **Your health depends on it.**

    This is a pretty obvious one, but it's amazing how we keep pushing our bodies thinking they will just be able to keep on going. Why is it that we treat our cars better than our bodies? Have you ever noticed that after a particularly stressful week of working long hours and feeling overwhelmed, you finally get to the weekend but wake up ill and can't leave the bed?

But then you feel guilty and force yourself to keep going because there are these things that need to be done. But how does that help you in the long run? The truth is, as I know only too well, that it really doesn't help at all.

Interestingly, if you don't put yourself first, your body will certainly kick in and force you to! Stress and lack of sleep take their toll on your body. They weaken your body's immune system and leave you more vulnerable to all sorts of nasty illnesses.

How many times have you ignored periods of illness and just kept working through them instead of taking the rest your body was asking for? Every time you have a major period of illness, the Universe is giving you the message to 'slow down'. You see, I used to ignore these sickness warnings and tried to keep going. The thing that I learnt is that if you ignore the occasions when the illness isn't too bad and keep going, a time will come when you will suffer a worse illness that is too serious to ignore. It will ensure that you cannot possibly get up and carry on working. It will force you to attend to the rest your body's needs.

So do start to listen to your body and honour its needs. You will truly reap the benefits in the long run.

3. **Your romantic relationships will flourish.**

   Whether you're in a relationship or looking for one, I guarantee that your partner will feel more enamoured with you and more fulfilled in the relationship when you're not afraid to make yourself a priority.

Firstly, by taking the necessary time for yourself, you give your partner the freedom to take that time for himself or herself. Everybody wins, and everybody's happy!

Secondly, when you're well rested and relaxed, you're much more fun to be around. You'll be less grumpy, irritable, and snappy. You will be able to deal with ups and downs in a calm and measured way.

It's all right if your partner misses you for a night because you need a yoga session and a bubble bath. The version of you that your partner gets afterwards is 10 times the partner your stressed-out self would be. So it really will be a win-win situation all round.

4. **Your friends and family will benefit.**

So you think your friends and family don't notice when they're talking to you and you're half asleep or mentally distracted? Think again. These people know you best and love you the most, and they would certainly much rather have you happy, healthy, and clearheaded when they see you. Yes, this is true even if it's a little less often because you needed to take some time for yourself! You'll be a better listener and more enjoyable to be around because you will be truly present with them.

You will also have fewer negative and difficult moments with your children, and you will be able to really enjoy special time with them too.

5. **You'll be happier, calmer, and more fulfilled.**

When you are at your happiest, you are most helpful to the world. We should all strive to be our happiest and do those things that make us happy, every day. Don't feel guilty about it; you are able to show up more for others when you start showing up for yourself first.

So don't be afraid to clear your schedule for a comforting and restorative massage, a yoga class, a walk in the park on your lunch break, or just a relaxing hot bath. Please don't be afraid to love yourself! After all, you are pretty amazing.

Take a minute now to tell yourself 'I am amazing'. Repeat it a few times, and say it out loud to yourself. Even better, stand in front of a mirror and look yourself in the eyes and say it several times, and truly mean it.

Action Step

So that you fully take on board and embody what you have been reading, I'd like you to take 10 minutes now and write down 5 things that you could start doing today to put yourself first.

Also, book out now an hour of 'me' time in your diary each week. Make this time sacrosanct so that you don't let anything else get in the way of that time. If you find the thought of booking out a whole hour for yourself a bit scary at the moment, then start booking just half an hour a week. Or make it two half hours a week. Then after a month, extend that to an hour.

2. Asking for Help

I don't know about you, but the message I was brought up to believe as a child was that if you couldn't do something on your own, then you were a failure. This has caused me to struggle and created a lot of stress in my life. That, to be honest with you,

I could quite easily have done without. It also meant that I put myself under no end of pressure as a result.

In addition, it meant that even if people offered to help me with something, I would say, 'Thank you' but turn it down. I used to find it very difficult to accept help from anybody most of the time.

But the reality is this: I would always be quick to offer help at all times to other people. It didn't matter if those individuals were friends, family, work colleagues, or even people I knew hardly at all. Why?

Well, it felt great to be able to help someone else out. It does, doesn't it?

So why do we deny other people that opportunity to feel great by helping us? It is really quite selfish behaviour.

You see, what I have learnt is that the most successful people in life don't get there by doing everything on their own. We have skills that we are good at, but there are many things that are not in our skill set. So trying to do things that we are really not any good at means that we spend an awful lot of time struggling. We get frustrated, and we stick at it for hours, and for what? What about the time we are wasting doing that?

We also have a tendency to get hung up on the fact that we may have to pay someone to do the task that we are not good at. We take the attitude that if we did it ourselves, it would be cheaper. But would it really? First of all, we tend not to put a value on our own time. So our time isn't worth anything. Really? Is that true?

If we are running our own business, we would charge out our time to a customer at an hourly rate. What might that hourly rate be, £10, £30, £50 per hour? So why in our personal lives do we not put an hourly rate on our time in the same way? The answer is that we do not see the worth of our own personal value.

In reality, if we struggle with things that are not in our skill set, we waste a lot of time. It is then quite likely that in the end, we don't actually do the job effectively, or we may actually give up somewhere along the line, irritated and frustrated with ourselves. I know this situation is very often the case when we are looking at making big changes in our lives.

I know that when I have asked people for help or invested in getting the help I needed, the end result was success rather than failure. I felt supported along the way. I had someone to ask questions to and to get answers, and the whole process was so much easier. I totally believe in 'success with ease' now. I no longer try and struggle on, but instead, I seek help from others when I know that it isn't a good use of my time to be doing something I don't like or am no good at. I let other people do what they love, and I get to do the same. That way, we both win.

3. Receiving Graciously

Have you ever been in a situation where someone expressed appreciation or gave you a compliment, and it embarrassed you or left you feeling a bit uncomfortable?

Think back to the last time someone complimented you. How did you respond?

If it was a compliment about what you were wearing, did you say, 'Thank you' and then say something like, 'Oh, it's just an old dress I've had for years'?

Did you quickly change the subject?

Or did you ignore it all together?

I always used to find it very uncomfortable when people paid me a compliment. I wasn't able to believe that they were saying those nice things about me. This was because I couldn't accept how anyone would actually think those good things about me. You know why? It's because I wouldn't accept believing those things about myself. I thought I wasn't worth it.

I also think that we feel people are just complimenting us because they feel they ought to, and consequently there is no real worth in it. There can be a belief that people give out compliments too easily and they are therefore not genuine. We may have a tendency to feel they are just trying to be nice rather than really meaning it. Most of the time, though, it is because we don't value ourselves enough to believe that other people want to say nice things about us.

Not receiving graciously can also be because we don't value the other person's opinion, we don't want to show vulnerability, or we have low self-esteem.

It is really important to learn and practice receiving compliments graciously. Do you know why? Receiving and giving compliments are good for your wellbeing. It releases endorphins (these cause a feel-good effect in your brain), and it raises your self-esteem and confidence. What better reason than this do you need to start practising the art of receiving and giving compliments?

If you have difficulty accepting and giving compliments, I would encourage you to think about why that might be the case. You see, when I was able to understand better why I was having difficulty accepting compliments, I was in a improved position to change my natural, habitual tendency.

If you find it difficult to receive a compliment, here are some tips on how to do it:

Firstly, all you need to do is just SMILE. This will show other people who are complimenting you that you welcome their thoughts. It will also help you to lift your energy.

Secondly, say 'Thank you, it is very nice of you to say that'. You are then showing the person that you value what he/she said.

Thirdly, you could then talk about why you are pleased to hear the compliment. If it's about a dress you are wearing, you could say things like, 'I really love wearing this dress because it makes me feel good' or 'It reminds me of a specific occasion that was really pleasurable', or 'I bought it when I was out with my 'friend X', and we had such fun that day'.

Action Step

The next time you hear a compliment, practice receiving it graciously using the steps listed above. After the person has paid you the compliment, just take a deep breath for a moment and receive it. You don't have to rush into a response. Then smile and say, 'Thank you'.

4. The Importance of Physical Exercise

Physical exercise is a very important part of keeping our bodies in great health. So it is good to get into a regular habit of doing exercise that raises your heart level and to stick at it.

I would encourage you to find something that you like doing, or even better, something that you love doing. If you choose something that you love, then you are going to continue to do it on a regular basis, and you will reap the rewards of improving the health and the physical tone of your body.

This exercise regime might include a yoga class, dancing, going to the gym, working with a personal trainer, Urban Rebounding, taking walks, swimming, or playing a sport. The choice is yours. Start to make it part of your regular life and part of your 'me' time.

Another option is to do one of these things with a friend. This way it is far more difficult to get out of doing it because you will be letting someone else down.

You will reap the best benefits and rewards to your health if you bring exercise in as a regular activity. A minimum would be to do something once a week, but if you can combine more than one activity a week, that would be more beneficial. For instance, you could combine swimming and then going out for walks in nature.

It is very important when losing weight to do some physical exercise along with the dietary changes. If you have not done any strenuous exercise for a long time, then I certainly would not recommend rushing headlong into long bouts of vigorous exercise. I would recommend that you talk to your doctor before embarking on an exercise program.

If you have done very little bodily training in the past, then I would just start with some very gentle exercises. Some simple movements working on your stomach muscles, for instance, can be done whilst you are still in bed. Another idea is to take yourself out for some gentle walks and increase the distance you go each week. You can also use the stairs instead of the lift or put on some music and dance.

As of today, I would encourage you to start putting yourself first and best. Remember what they tell you to do in the case of an emergency when you are on an aeroplane. Put your oxygen mask first. If you don't start making your health a priority, you won't always be able to be there for your family. By putting yourself first, you are ensuring that you will show up as the best version of yourself for your family.

Access your Free bonuses at www.loveyourgutbook.com

CHAPTER 10

Keep Your Motor Running

'All you need is the plan, the road map, and the courage to press on to your destination'.

—Earl Nightingale

THE MOST IMPORTANT THING IS that you are going to start this journey to ecstatic health for you and yourself alone. You are going to do this because you are fed up with feeling tired all the time. You are sick of being unhealthy and not being able to do all things in life that you really want to do. You definitely want to take your life to a new level and free yourself from being stuck and repeating the same old patterns.

The problem is that you can't keep on doing the same old things and expect to get a different result. It just doesn't work that way. Once you make the decision to take control of your health, then other things will start to shift in your life for the better.

If you have children, wouldn't it be great to set them the

example of how to be eating healthfully? You can show them how important it is to put yourself first and be the best for your family. You will also be showing them how you value yourself and your health. When you do that for yourself, you can help them to look after their own health so that when they are adults and are getting older, their health will be in a much better place than if they don't take care.

Eating healthfully from a young age is an investment for good health in your later years. It is also never too late to start taking control or your health.

Dealing with Well-Meaning but Unhelpful Comments

So you have made that decision to take control of your health and follow the process in outlined in this book. You then may tell your partner, some of your friends, or your family members, and you will start to get some well-meaning but often unhelpful comments.

I would recommend that you do not go into detail about the eating plan you will be following. The reason I say this is because you will get comments from people who are not going to help you to stay on track and see this through to the end. Everyone will have their own version of why you shouldn't be doing it. The comments from other people, however, will merely reflect their own fears. You need to bear that in mind. Their comments will be coming from a place of well-meaning, but they won't be helpful to you.

So I would be ready to thank people for their advice, but tell them that you are absolutely fine. People will be coming from a place of good intentions, but their comments could sabotage you. Yet you need to stay strong in your belief that you really want to take control of your health and step into the new healthy, energised you. Be proud of the decision you have made. It takes a lot of courage to make a change in your life like this.

You are going to love it at the end when they all start saying, 'Wow! Gosh, you are looking healthy, slimmer, and more vibrant!'

Creating a Daily Routine

It will be really important for you to create a daily routine for yourself. This will help to make the transition to a new way of eating and a new way of living your life so much easier. It will also ensure that you really get the most benefit from this process.

The key thing to remember is that getting organised and planned in advance will make things so much easier for you to stick to the new way of eating. Make sure that you always have snacks such as nuts (almonds and pecans) as well as some Crunchy Munchy Seeds available. Particularly do this when you are going out for the day. Also, make sure that you carry a bottle of filtered or mineral water with you as well.

Create a list of all of the things that you need to do each day. Start from when you wake up in the morning, which would include things like your regular meditation time, drinking hot water and lemon as the first drink of the day, and listing out the vitamins, minerals, and other supplements that you need take with their dosage for each week. That way, it will be easier to remember, and you will soon get into the habit of doing all the things that you need to do.

Speak kindly to yourself every day, and if you slip up in any way, don't beat yourself up, but just take the experience as a learning experience and move on. Whilst you are on this journey, you are going to find that there will be ups and downs. There will be physical and emotional things that will come up, but don't let these challenges take you off track. The end result will definitely be worth some of the ups and downs.

Just be aware that you may find a return of the cravings for sugar and carbohydrates when you start to take the caprylic acid at the start of Week 6, but it shouldn't last for more than a few days. Just make sure that you reach out for a glass of filtered or mineral water first. Then if you need to, you can nibble on some healthy snacks such as the Crunchy Munchy Seeds or the pecan and almond nuts. You could also check back to the written tips in dealing with sugar and carbohydrate cravings in Chapter 5 and follow those.

Make sure that you have the support of a friend or your partner so that if anything gets difficult, you have someone to turn to and provide that support to keep on track. Just remember, you are not a failure if you ask for help. Successful people ask for help.

Keeping Hydrated

One of the most important things is to ensure that you keep your body fully hydrated all the time. If drinking water on a regular basis is not something that you have been terribly good at before, then I would recommend some of the following tips to help you keep regularly hydrated.

Tip 1

Make sure that you put a jug of filtered or mineral water on your desk together with a glass the first thing in the morning. Then ensure that you keep drinking and regularly filling up throughout the day. You should aim to drink at least 2 pints in the morning. Then, at lunchtime, I recommend that you refill the jug so that it lasts you throughout the afternoon. You will notice that when you start to increase your hydration on a regular basis, your ability to focus and concentrate will start to improve.

Tip 2

If you are busy doing chores at home or working in the garden, I would recommend that you set a reminder on your phone so that you you don't forget to drink on a regular basis. Setting a reminder every hour would be a useful thing to do.

Tip 3

Make sure that when you go out, you take a bottle of filtered/ mineral water with you. This way you will ensure that you continue to drink regularly even though you are out.

Tip 4

Drinking a pint of water before you leave home every morning is a good way to ensure that you arrive at work fully hydrated and ready to be highly productive.

Don't Skip Breakfast

Breakfast is one of the most important meals of the day. I would highly recommend that you make sure to always have breakfast. Take advantage of some of the quick ways to prepare breakfasts listed in Chapter 6 to make certain that you always do this. If you feel that you don't have time for breakfast in the morning, then start to get into the habit of getting up earlier to allow yourself time to do it. Make healthful eating and looking after your body a priority. It is extremely important, and your body will thank you for it. You will also notice that you will be more effective in the morning at work.

Plan Ahead

By getting into the habit of planning and scheduling your meals ahead, you will start to change your mindset. You will change from feeling too busy to eat properly to wanting to honour your body, feed it, and nourish it with good, healthful, natural food.

We all have just 24 hours in the day. The difference is choosing to make and prioritise the time to look after your body by feeding it well and ensuring good health. By doing that on a regular basis, you will find that you waste less time procrastinating, and you will actually become more productive. This is because your body and mind will both be functioning at a much more effective level.

Bring in Exercise as Part of Your Health

Please don't forget that regular exercise is very important for your overall health and wellbeing. So plan it into your weekly schedule and make it sacrosanct. Also, choose to do the type of exercise that you love. Then you are likely to stick to it and make it a regular routine.

Follow the 90-Day Process

By following the 90-day process as outlined in this book and following Your Ecstatic Health Eating plan and sticking to it, you will realise a change in your overall health and energy and a reduction in your weight. In order to help you to do that, I have summarised below the key stages in the program, but this does not encompass all of the details. Therefore, I would encourage you to read the book again. Get yourself a notepad and pen too so that you can note down all of the key things you need to do to ensure that you do not miss anything.

1. Make the decision that you are committed to wanting the end result.

2. Do the exercise in Chapter One, and create the vision of what you want to see for yourself at the end of this 90-day journey.

3. Review your food storage cupboard and fridge, and clear out any foods that should not be eaten or are old, out of date, or mouldy.

4. Review the shopping list and tick off anything that you already have that is current and in date. Make a list of all the things you need to buy, including food products and natural supplements. You can leave the caprylic acid and grapefruit seed extract until week 5. But buy the things you need that are on your shopping list.

5. Measure and weigh yourself and log these on 'Your Ecstatic Health Body Profile' at www. loveyourgutbook.com. Get someone to take a photograph of you as you are now.

6. Start your Week 1 and 2 winding-down process by reducing your consumption of the foods that will no longer be serving you as you start on Your Ecstatic Health Eating Plan.

7. Access your free bonuses at www.loveyourgutbook. com.

8. Start writing down the physical and emotional changes you are experiencing in 'Your Ecstatic Health Journal'.

9. Start meditating with the free bonus guided meditation that is available at www.loveyourgutbook. com.

10. Start the daily dry skin brushing process to help your body rid itself of toxins.

11. In Week 2, plan out your menu for the next week, and make a shopping list of things that you will need for your meals. You will be starting to eat on **Your Ecstatic Health Eating Plan**™ in the next week.

12. In Week 3, start following **Your Ecstatic Health Eating Plan**™ for all of your meals.

13. Follow the tips to help with any detox symptoms that you might start to feel. If you follow these and drink lots of filtered or mineral water, it will only last for 2 or 3 days.

14. Start bringing in the TLC into your life. Plan time into your diary every week for you to do what you love. Also, start spending time at the end of each day writing down the things you are grateful for.

15. If you currently do very little or no exercise, then start to gently introduce some into your day and week. You need to keep it going on a regular basis. Then build up slowly to doing more each week.

I wish you every success on your journey to a more vibrant, healthy, and slimmer you and life. **Just remember to put yourself first, and you will be putting yourself best!**

Should you feel that you need some support on this journey, then there are ways that you can get it. You can find out more at www.loveyourgutbook.com.

'Hi Sue—just saw my before and after photos! OMG! Now I see why you're so pleased! I cannot believe my eyes! Such a difference—mostly my face and change to the look in my eyes is startling! To be honest, I think I've been brought back from the brink! Heartfelt thanks to you. You truly are an earth angel. Bless you for the work you are doing'.

—Julie xx

46231397R00075

Made in the USA
Charleston, SC
13 September 2015